# Goodbye Obesity

# Goodbye Obesity

**KISS OBESITY GOODBYE AND SAY HELLO TO HOLISTIC WELLNESS**

Jean D. François MD

**Other books written by Dr. Jean Daniel François:**

*Les Clés de la réussite* (Edition Parole, Québec, Canada, 2008)

*The No-Nonsense Approach to a Successful Life* (Xulon Press, USA, 2008)

*Prescription for a Successful Life* (New York, 2010)

*Prescription for a Successful Career in Medicine* (New York, 2010)

*Prescription for an Exciting Love Life* (New York, 2010)

*Through the Light of Sola Scriptura (À la Lumière de Sola Scriptura)* (New York, 2010)

*Les contours de l'Amour (On the Edge of Love)* (New York, 2011)

*On the Path of SOLA FIDE (Sur le Sentier de SOLA FIDE)* (Tait Publishing Company, U.S.A, 2013)

*La santé Au Bout de vos Doigts* (New York, 2012)

*Your Health at Your Fingertips* (New York, 2017)

*ESCAPADE: A Collection of Poems in French Covering the Various Aspects of Life* (Les éditions Persée, France, 2017)

You may visit the author's website at www.prescriptionfo-rasuccessfullife.com.

On the other hand, you may write, e-mail, or call with questions, comments, or requests:

Jean Daniel François, 1713-19 Ralph Avenue, Brooklyn, NY 11236

Phone: 718-531-6100
Fax: 718-531-2329
E-mail: jfranc6704@aol.com

# Acknowledgments

Writing a book on health is a huge undertaking that requires the collaboration of a distinguished team. I cannot compose the imposing list of all those who have helped me. I am afraid I may run the risk of omitting a few names. I can safely state that this book is made possible because of the contribution and encouragement of many people. I want to thank them all. However, Dr. Susan Tree, EdD, RD, CDN, is one person who stands out in countless ways, including spending hours upon hours reading and reviewing the manuscript, providing very useful expert advice until the end. I am eternally grateful to her.

I would like to express my special gratitude to my daughter, Sarah J. François, for her dedication, her commitment, and her resourcefulness. She enthusiastically took the book and freely made corrections, rearranged it, and provided insights to make sure it is reader friendly. Therefore, this book is also dedicated to her and to all the other outstanding contributors.

Overall, I am grateful to you, the readers who are committed to learning and making changes to improve your health. I tip my hat to you. I wish you all the best on your journey to learn or review the information needed for you to stay healthy and combat obesity.

# Disclaimer

The information contained in this book is provided only for the reader's general health education and guidance. It does not intend to replace the role of anyone's physician or any other competent professional who assists in securing a healthy life. Specific comments regarding symptoms, diagnosis, prescriptions, prognosis, treatment options, and other individual medical recommendations must come from a competent physician after appropriate thorough examination. This book is based on the professional and personal experience and observations of a medical professional. It is another approach to remind or to highlight ideas that can benefit and educate an astute reader who is seriously engaged in the journey for a healthier and more meaningful life. Do not ignore advice from your qualified health-care provider and pharmaceutical or nutritionist advisers. If you do not have a physician, seek a reliable one. The author will not be held responsible or judged liable to anyone or institution for any loss, disappointment, or damage attributed directly or indirectly by the ideas expressed in this book. Any examples and any names used do not represent any specific individuals or institutions. Feel free to contact me with any questions or comments to inform me of any error that may have inadvertently slipped in. Thanks!

# Table of Contents

Acknowledgments · · · · · · · · · · · · · · · · · · · · · · ·vii

Disclaimer · · · · · · · · · · · · · · · · · · · · · · · · · · · · ix

Foreword · · · · · · · · · · · · · · · · · · · · · · · · · · · · ·xv

Part I        The Challenge of Obesity · · · · · · · · · · · · · · · ·1

Chapter 1     What Is Obesity? · · · · · · · · · · · · · · · · · · · · · ·3

Chapter 2     Obesity in History · · · · · · · · · · · · · · · · · · · · ·9

Chapter 3     Causes of Obesity · · · · · · · · · · · · · · · · · · · · ·14

Chapter 4     Consequences of Being Obese · · · · · · · · · · ·38

Chapter 5      Eleven Myths Regarding Overweight
               and Obesity ·······························43

Chapter 6      The Peculiarity of Obesity················52

Chapter 7      Why Is Obesity So Prevalent?············57

Part II        How to Face the Challenge of Obesity····65

Chapter 8      Deciphering the Yo-Yo Phenomenon
               of Weight Loss and Gain ················67

Chapter 9      The Dieting Approach in
               Addressing Obesity······················80

Chapter 10     Physical Activities to Tackle Obesity···· 106

Chapter 11     Combating Obesity:
               Bullets to Load Your Gun ·············· 113

Chapter 12     Role of Medication and
               Surgery in Treating Obesity ············ 131

Chapter 13     Facing the Challenge of the
               Weight-Loss Plateau ··················· 143

Chapter 14　Keeping Obesity at Bay for Good······· 150

Chapter 15　Food for Thought······················· 163

Chapter 16　Children and Obesity ··················· 173

Epilogue······························· 183

About the Author ····················· 185

Selected Bibliography················· 187

Other Useful Sources ················· 189

# Foreword

By now, most of us are aware of the alarming data regarding the percentage of the population that is overweight or obese. This is the reason why most people are paying attention to their weight and want to identify ways to reduce its prevalence. Even the most skeptical people want to switch gears and focus on ways to stay fit and enjoy life. Unfortunately, the ultimate goal may be obvious, but the road leading to it is often murky. We are bombarded with so much information; we are being pulled in so many different directions, that at times we feel trapped in a maze. This is why I decided to write this book, *Good-Bye, Obesity*. The goals of *Good-Bye, Obesity* aim to provide the following:

1. The various causes for overweight and obesity and why they have reached such a proportion

2. Simple, down-to-earth steps to address them individually and collectively
3. Tools for each reader to determine where he or she stands
4. Ways and means to overcome the plateau
5. Ways to keep the weight off and stay healthy and fit

Overall, weight control remains a serious challenge for all. I want each reader to know what is at stake and to empower him or her to take the necessary actions to engage on the road for a healthy and long life. To reach such a goal, this book is easily accessible and affordable. I would like all readers to be able to change the way they look and feel. Let this be your kick start to health.

Finally, the success of this book depends not only on the number of readers but on the number of people who choose to act on what they know, practice what they learn or are reminded of, and are willing and ready to fight the winnable fight to grow old healthy and fit. Ultimately, every one of us is in charge of our health! I know that together we can do it. I thank you, and I congratulate you in advance!

*The body is a ship which must not be overloaded.*
—Plutarch, Greek historian

# PART I

## The Challenge of Obesity

# CHAPTER 1

## What Is Obesity?

I n the twenty-first century, our world faces a countless number of challenges. Health issues in general and obesity in particular figure among some of the top worries. Obesity has become a growing worldwide concern. This pandemic affects all age groups, all classes, and all races.

From its Latin origin *obesitas*, obesity is defined as an increase in the body weight, a condition in which there is an excess accumulation of body fat to the extent that it can compromise one's health condition and overall life expectancy. There is an imbalance between the number of calories consumed that exceeds the amount of calories burned. In other words, it is eating too much while not being active enough to burn at least all the calories taken in during the meals. Obviously, such a definition is by far too simplistic because there are multiple other factors that affect weight. This will be explained in further detail on the following pages.

Obesity is determined by a measurement called *body mass index* (BMI). The BMI formula is the result of the work done by Belgium statistician Adolphe Quetelet (1796–1874). It was initially called the "Quetelet Index." BMI is used internationally to measure obesity. It is a measure of body fat based on one's height and weight and is determined by dividing the person's weight in kilograms by the square of his or her height in meters ($kg/m^2$).

### BMI Weight Status Categories

| BMI | Weight Status |
|---|---|
| Below 18.5 | Underweight |
| 18.5–24.9 | Normal |
| 25.0–29.9 | Overweight |
| 30.0 and above | Obese |
| 40.0 and above | Morbidly Obese |

## The Steps Leading Up to Obesity

According to experts, a person with a desirable weight for height has a BMI between 18.5 and 25. Further research suggests that other factors should be taken into consideration, including age (a higher BMI seems to be desirable in the elderly), gender, "big bones," a high percentage of muscle, fluid retention (edema), and loss of limbs (amputation). These factors can make the BMI measurement inaccurate. There are also other measures of obesity, including waist circumference, which measures fat accumulated around the abdomen. A man's waist should be less than forty inches, and a woman's ideal waist should not go beyond thirty-four to thirty-five inches. The waist-to-hip ratio (WHR) for men should be less than 0.9 and women less than 0.8 to be considered healthy. There is also a newer and more accurate measure of healthy weight: the waist to height ratio (WHtR). It is the waist circumference divided by the height and should be less than 0.5 for men and women. Nevertheless, whenever the body fat accumulated to the point of having a BMI between twenty-five and thirty $kg/m^2$, WHR of more than 1.0, and WHtR of more than 0.5, one has become **overweight** (the weight is more than the ideal weight) and needs to take steps toward gradual weight loss. If the trend continues, one can become clinically obese, leading to many associated health concerns

## Obesity

Although there is a general tendency to use the word *obesity* loosely, it is recommended that we make the difference between those who are plainly obese and those who are overweight. If someone has a BMI of 30 $kg/m^2$ or more, he or she is considered obese. A BMI between 25 and 29.9 is classified as overweight. One can be categorized as severely obese, morbidly obese, or super obese. It may sound paradoxical, but obesity does not necessarily mean being well nourished. Actually, it is often a sign of malnutrition because the adopted food regimen is not healthy and does not have the proper micronutrients. The excess fat can hide a low muscle mass.

Obesity has become an epidemic. This means it is occurring in proportion beyond the level of normal expectancy. In many instances, it is not a benign condition. According to the World Health Organization (WHO), obesity has more than doubled since 1980. Obesity and overweight are the fifth leading risk of global death. "In 2014, more than 1.9 billion adults, 18 years and older, were overweight. Of these over 600 million were obese. 39% of adults aged 18 years and over were overweight in 2014, and 13% were obese. Most of the world's population lives in countries where overweight and obesity kills more people than underweight. 41 million children under the age of 5 were overweight or obese in 2014."[1]

Overweight and obesity are related to 2.8 million adults' deaths annually along with other conditions such as more than 40 percent of diabetes, almost 25 percent

---

1  WHO, Obesity and overweight fact sheet. Updated June 2016.

of coronary heart disease, and an increased percentage of certain cancers.

From the United States to Asia and Europe, the prevalence of obesity is increasing. According to the WHO, obesity has more than doubled since 1980. Globally, around 35 percent of adults ages twenty and older were overweight in 2008. According to the National Institutes of Health (NIH), in the United States, more than two-thirds of the adult population is either overweight or obese, more than one-third are just obese, and more than one in twenty adults are considered to be extremely obese. As far as children are concerned, about one-third of children and adolescents ages six to nineteen meet the criteria to be classified as overweight or obese; more than one in six children and adolescents ages six to nineteen are obese. Among Hispanics and black people, the numbers are even higher in America. If the experts are right, in a couple years or so, the number of people who are overweight will reach more than two billion adults and the number of people obese more than seven hundred million. [2]

BMI may also be affected by weight and muscle mass. A well-built athlete is likely to have an elevated BMI not necessarily due to fat but to increased muscle mass. The BMI number is to be considered a tool. One should not

---

2  National Institutes of Health, "Clinical guidelines on the identification, evaluation, and treatment of overweight and obesity in adults: The evidence report." National Heart, Lung, and Blood Institute; September 1998. NIH Publication No. 98–4083. ww.nhibi.nih.gov/NIH.

only pay attention to BMI but preferably to overall medical profile, gender, age, muscular condition, and ethnic background.

The annual death toll due to obesity in the United States is in the hundreds of thousands. Unless there is a change in the current trend, the number will keep climbing. It is the fifth leading risk for global deaths and raises the cost of health care for obese people.

The *financial aspect* of obesity cannot be underestimated. On the one hand, the weight-loss industry that keeps offering products and services to lose or control weight generates more than $40 billion; on the other hand, those who are obese and have associated health complications cost close to $170 billion annually. This is a challenge and burden for everyone.

# CHAPTER 2

## Obesity in History

Throughout history, obesity has been perceived in several different ways. For example, before the twentieth century, obese women were considered beautiful and elegant. Today, magazines feature stick-thin models as the standard for beauty and forward fashion. In the beginning, people strove to look like goddesses such as Venus, Aphrodite, and Isis. Then changes in culture caused the standard of beauty to shift. History reports that it was Egypt and China who first raised the concern that obesity affects health negatively.

The perception of obesity has shifted back and forth depending on geographic region and time. In some countries, until recently, obesity was still viewed as a sign of prosperity. Furthermore, having some extra layers of fat was considered by some as a source of insulation to protect against weather conditions and famine.

It was also rumored to aid with fertility. Many books and thousands of poems were written to celebrate women with curves. We see it in the arts, the museums, and our literature.[3]

Not too long ago in certain geographic regions, overweight people represented the elite upper class and a better social status. They symbolized wealth, abundance, and opulence and were the envy of the rest of the population. In those regions, a person who was light or skinny was considered weak, sickly, and in need of a better health regime. There were even people who bought extra padding to put in their clothes or took medications to boost their appetites to gain weight. Obesity does not mean the same to everyone everywhere. Nevertheless, because of globalization, the trend is quickly changing worldwide.

There are also special circumstances that change perception of weight standards. For example, chubby babies are usually perceived as healthy and well cared for. Even now, people consider babies with round faces to look adorable. Small, skinny babies imply signs of malnourishment or being unhealthy.

By the nineteenth century, obesity had become less desirable. Many government agencies began to address

---

3  Haslam, David, and Neville Rigby, "A long look at obesity," *The Lancet.* Vol. 376, no. 9735, p. 85–86, 10 July 2010.

the appropriate proportion of fats, proteins, and carbo-hydrates in a balanced diet. The life-insurance industry started to provide guidelines for healthy insurers. This was the start of the food group age.

In 1916, the US Department of Agriculture made pub-lic the five food groups. Within the film and fashion indus-tries, people were exhibiting more glamorous figures with more skin and legs exposed, and the well-rounded figure was making room for people to flaunt their beauty—the taste and perception of beauty kept adjusting.

During the World War II period, some declarations on ideal weight in proportion to height were made available. Obesity was no longer fashionable or attractive. The expo-sition of larger bodies or chubby faces was no longer the norm. There was a craving for fitness and the advent of the dieting craze. It became fashionable to be slim. Stars such as Betty Grable, Marilyn Monroe, and Jayne Mansfield were admired for their contours and their curvy shapes.

By the second half of the twentieth century and into the twenty-first century, there was a standard body, face, hairstyle, outfit, and way to walk that was established as the new archetype to strive for.

In the twenty-first century, obesity has become an epidemic in many parts of the globe. Here is what the WHO declared in its press release of 2003: "Obesity is a complex condition, one with serious social and psychological dimensions, that affects virtually all ages and socioeconomic groups and threatens to overwhelm both developed and developing countries. In 1995, there were an estimated 200 million obese adults worldwide and another 18 million children under five classified as overweight. As of 2000, the number of obese adults has increased to over 300 million. Contrary to conventional wisdom, the obesity epidemic is not restricted to industrialized societies; in developing countries, it is estimated that over 115 million people suffer from obesity-related problems."[4]

Nowadays, the most popular stars and models seem to set the trend when it comes to beauty and fitness. They catch the gaze of everyone. They define the norm, what is acceptable, and what is expected. From the nineteenth century forward, our culture has become more and more favorable toward being slim and sexy. Furthermore, with the advent of so much technology, many people want to live the lavish life of the stars and the models who are slim and glamorous.

There is currently a campaign against obesity. Yet at least one out of nine people remain obese. Our mass media images do not seem to help with our national and

---

4 Ecknoyan, Garabed, "A History of Obesity, or How What Was Good Became Ugly and Then Bad." Vol. 13, iss. 4, pp. 421–427, October 2006. WHO, "Controlling the global obesity epidemic." ACKDJournal.org.

international obesity struggle. Why is there this dichoto-my between what the ideal body type is and our current state of affairs?

# CHAPTER 3

## Causes of Obesity

**Diet**

One of the causes of being overweight or obese has to do with the quantity and the quality of foods we eat. Obesity occurs when the number of calories consumed is greater than the amount used by the body. There is a remaining surplus of calories that causes excessive fat accumulation. If such a process continues, more fat accumulates and will likely have an adverse effect on health. For those of us who are living in developed nations where we have a lot of food available, we tend to consume more than the portion needed. As a result, a high percentage of our population tends to get fat because we overeat.

In addition, the quality of our food has also changed. We tend to consume a lot of animal fats; however, because of the proven heart disease risk of *trans*-fatty acids (used mainly in processed food, often baked goods), trans fats have been banned, and manufacturers have replaced them with other fats and energy-dense micronutrients. These are poor meals while we decrease the consumption of legumes, fruits, vegetables, whole grains, and nuts. The FDA has taken steps to better our diets, starting with the ban on trans fats—but is it enough? We tend to have increased intake of salt, fat, and sugar. The current typical diet in many instances is composed of an all-you-can-eat buffet with steak, shrimp, lobster, chicken, some fish, carbohydrates, and large sugary drinks throughout the meal. The popular diet is made up of highly refined, processed foods high in fat, calories, salt, and sugars, with decreased amounts of vitamins and minerals. These meals are consumed quickly and conveniently and in large portions with the privilege to get another plate with the same types of foods. If you are like the people of the new generation, you will likely top off your meal with large scoops of ice cream and cake. To be fair, sometimes these people will also consume a few leaves of lettuce and a diet soda. Next time, check the amount of salt in that burger when you visit a fast-food or chain restaurant and perhaps rethink dessert.

Oversized, high-calorie fast foods and sweetened drinks are easily accessible and cheaper than the healthier fruit and vegetables. In some neighborhoods, you simply cannot find a fresh fruit or vegetable anywhere. However, when we eat whatever is available, and it tastes good, our taste buds form an affinity for having those types of foods. If something looks good, smells good, and tastes good, we are likely to want to eat it. Immediately after eating these types of foods, we sometimes feel tired and sluggish. Sometimes, we go so far as to sleep immediately after consuming a large amount of food, which is definitely not optimal for health.

We are ready to resume the same trend day in and out, and it becomes a vicious cycle that we cannot break. Some of us would not have it any other way though—we enjoy this lifestyle of ours. In our minds, we start associating food with "rewarding ourselves" for the hard work we put in daily in our generally stressful environments. Perhaps this is where the term *comfort food* comes from.

Our way of eating has changed during the last few decades. Because of economic strains and changes in family structure, both parents may be working, fewer people have time to cook, and many people do not know how to cook anymore. In recent years, there has been less of an emphasis on sit-down family meals as most of us are constantly on the go and "too busy." We thus begin to eat out more. For breakfast, lunch, or dinner, we go to restaurants, coffee shops, fast-food locales, and vending machines or street vendors that are convenient to appease or satisfy our hunger. We consume what is tasty and attractive but not necessarily the healthiest. To make matters worse, in some neighborhoods, people do not have easy access to places where they can buy healthier foods to change their diets.

## Environment

For our purposes, environment is defined as eating habits, types of physical activities, and types of community we are exposed to. Because our genes are not modified or changed overnight, environment plays an important role when considering obesity. From the second part of the twentieth century, the population's eating habits and level of activities have changed considerably. For example, we have become more dependent on fast-food consumption. We have become more complacent while adopting a sedentary lifestyle and enjoying the latest "labor-saving devices" invented to make us more comfortable and alleviate our burdens. As a result, we have decreased our amount of physical activities. Cars have taken the place of bikes. Getting a Starbucks coffee seems easier than eating a bowl of cereal before leaving home. We have also become happier in front of the screen, especially children.

Before going any further, let us point out that *physical activity* is defined as any body movement that requires the use of our skeletal muscles. Whether it is walking, biking, swimming, running, or dancing, such a movement causes energy expenditure that does not occur during inactivity. It is reported that globally, 6 percent of deaths occur because of physical inactivity. The current, more sedentary life accounts for five million deaths every year. According to WHO data, physical inactivity also plays a significant role in diseases such as breast and colon cancers, ischemic heart disease, cerebrovascular disease, hormonal imbalance, and diabetes. While we enjoy all the new devices such as remote-control TVs, washing machines, elevators, dishwashers, computers, Internet, iPhones, and video games, we must realize that they also encourage a couch-potato lifestyle.

As part of our modern way of living, we no longer walk to neighborhood stores. There is an increasing amount of sedentary work with long hours that require less use of physical strength. With improved modes of transportation and the societal changes mentioned above, we have become an overall more sedentary society. Now when most of us go into work, we sit at our desks, stand periodically, and click buttons on a screen; most of the time, we barely have to get up. I can order a pizza for lunch right from my laptop. Whereas before we had to walk or bike long distances to get somewhere, now we merely exercise our right ankles when we have to halt our personal vehicles. Furthermore, even for those who desire to be more active, our places of work or school are such a great distance away from our homes, they require us to drive or take mass transit.

At times, there is no safe way to walk, ride, or run from point A to point B. For example, there are neighborhoods where you would be hard pressed to find a sidewalk. In those neighborhoods, you are walking at your risk. Other neighborhoods have no gyms, no recreation centers, no parks, no playgrounds, and no affordable public transportation. If there are any gathering places, they tend to be bars and places to play video games, watch TV, or just hang out.

Even sweating has become unacceptable. The standard is that we must be clean and good smelling at all times, which is why some people go through great pains to carry travel deodorant and a toothbrush and toothpaste in their work bags. For some of us, the extent of exercise is surfing the net or watching our favorite sports. In other words, we exercise our eyes and our hands rather than our bodies

If we remain active, in addition to cutting down or consuming within our estimated range of calories, we can lose weight or maintain our current weights—all other factors being equal. The body will start depleting fat storage as its primary source of energy. When we stay active, it tames our appetites somewhat because we are focused on other priorities, and we tend to feel better about ourselves. Staying active also increases our metabolisms as calories are being expended. Of course, the process of obesity is much more complex than just that. Other factors need to be considered.

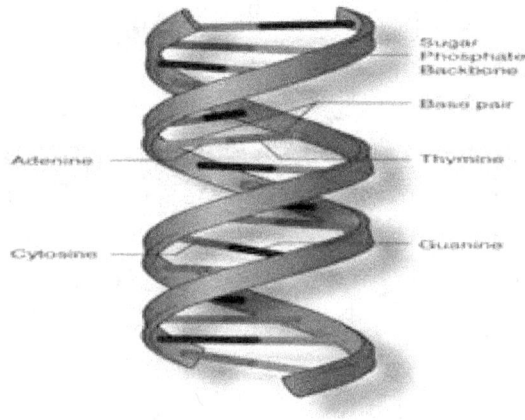

Google: DNA double helix picture

## Genetic Influences

There is a widely held belief that genetics play a role in who becomes obese. Obviously, not all of us who consume excessive amounts of food become overweight or obese. In fact, we may have friends who consume twice as much food as we do and remain thin. We bristle at the unfairness of such a circumstance. Alas! No one can choose his or her genes.

It is not uncommon to observe that many members of our immediate families are either thin or obese. Studies have been done that include twins, siblings, and family by adoption and their relation to obesity. These studies reveal how children tend to have the weights and shapes that are closer to their biological parents than to their adoptive parents. Two-thirds of children with obese parents who have been obese since childhood are likely to become obese; the same is true for those who are slim. This supports the fact that genes do have an effect on our shapes, our way of storing and distributing fat, and our metabolisms. Not only are we genetically predisposed to being thin or overweight but certain populations are also at higher risk of developing chronic illnesses such as diabetes even if they are thin.

Unfortunately, some of us are more genetically predisposed to develop obesity than others. We have to face facts. Accepting who we are and where we come from can go a long way in our approach to handling this condition. Perhaps our own improved health may spur others in our family to action too.

Researchers believe that there are more than four hundred genes associated with obesity. The effect of genetics in predisposing us to obesity is felt not only on our metabolic rates and ability to process fats, but it also involves our brains' ability -for example- to make us experience—through the hypothalamic pathways—hunger and satiety and therefore affect our behavior toward the amount and the quality of food we intake. This may shed light on the difference in how people respond when in the same environment and exposed to the same variables. Studies also reveal that if the people who are genetically predisposed to become obese take the appropriate steps, when placed in the proper environment, they are able to lose weight and keep the pounds off. So just because your whole family is obese, it does not mean you should give up hope.

In addition, there are a few other factors that independently affect obesity: age, gender, and body shape. It is documented that as we go through the aging process, we tend to become less active and less likely to exercise, and our aerobic capacity goes down. We may even lose some of our muscle mass, and metabolism slows. Therefore, unless we decrease our food intake, remain consciously active, and add variety and increase the amount of time and intensity of our exercise, we are likely to gain weight, especially as we become middle aged. Where the fat accumulates is also important. Having a pear-shaped body rather than an apple-shaped body (where the fat has accumulated in the middle abdomen area) is thought to be better.

In terms of gender, a woman's rate of metabolism is slower than that of a man's, especially after menopause. It is more difficult for women to lose or maintain their weight, while men tend to burn calories much more easily. Depending on our body shapes and our genders (BMI, adiposity), we may be more or less susceptible to weight variations. Because children tend to follow the habits and lifestyles of their parents, children of obese parents have an increased chance of becoming obese themselves. Of course, we do not want to have our children at a disadvantage at such an early age in life. Therefore, as parents, we have the ability to influence and mold our children's relationships with food and other activities that can positively affect their health choices.

## DNA Methylation

Among the causes of obesity, scientists agree that although it is multifactorial, genetic and environmental factors play an important role in such a disease. New research points out: that DNA methylation, which is a mechanism used by cells to control gene expression, [5] is another link contributing to obesity. As a matter of fact, significant changes have been identified in DNA methylation's role as a contributing factor in obesity". Study reveals - for exemple - "Hypocaloric-diet-induced weight loss in humans could alter DNA methylation status of specific genes. Moreover, baseline DNA methylation patterns may be used as epigenetic markers that could help to predict weight loss".[6] There is quite a number of studies that are exploring the changes in DNA methylation in relation to weight reduction / variation. The role of DNA methylation in various diseases. Emerging research also points out the key role of DNA methylation in regulating cellular differentiation. Overall, this is another avenue with new opportunities for the scientific community to help us better understand the complicated notion of obesity.

5  Mendelson M. M., R.E. Marioni, R. Joehanes, et al., "Association of Body Mass Index with DNA Methylation and Gene Expression in Blood Cells and Relations to Cardiometabolic Disease: A Mendelian Randomization Approach." *PLOS Medicine.* Accessed January 17, 2017. http://journals.plos.org/plosmedicine/article?id=10.1371/journal.pmed.1002215.
CL Relton, A Groom, B St Pourcain, *et al.***DNA methylation patterns in cord blood DNA and body size in childhood**
PLoS One, 7 (2012), p. e31821

6  **The Federation of American Societies for Experimental Biology, A dual epigenomic approach for the search of obesity biomarkers: DNA methylation in relation to diet-induced weight loss, Published online before printJanuary 5, 2011, doi:10.1096/fj.10-170365April 2011The FASEB Journalvol. 25 no. 4 1378-1389**

## Biochemical and Medical Ailments

Any medical condition causing little or no mobility can contribute to obesity. Certain medical conditions such as hypothyroidism, arthritis, polycystic ovarian syndrome, and Cushing disease can have a significant role for some people in weight gain through water accumulation, decreased or no mobility, or other mechanism. Certain medications like steroids, antidepressants, mood stabilizers, and others can also provide a favorable milieu for obesity. This does not mean that you should abruptly stop taking your psychiatric medication. This merely means that if you were concerned about weight gain and taking said medications, it would be a good idea to have a frank dialogue with your physician.

## Hormonal Changes

Even though the whole world is concerned about obesity rates, we have not been able to pinpoint every single cause and address those causes globally as well as individually. However, until a research study counters this, we can assume that if the exchange between calories used and consumed, the types of foods, the lifestyle, and the level of physical activity play their roles in contributing to obesity, then hormonal imbalances also may play a part.

Within our bodies, there are a handful of small glands that handle bodily functions by releasing the appropriate hormones for certain tasks. These parts of the body—the pancreas, adrenal glands, testes, ovaries, thyroid, parathyroid, thymus, hypothalamus, pituitary gland, and pineal gland—secrete chemical substances that work as messengers circulating throughout our tissues and organs. The secreted hormones are vital for the smooth functioning at various levels for the well-being of our bodies. A lack or a surplus of certain kinds of hormones may trigger a handful of health conditions and may even lead to death.

It is worth pointing out that not all the hormones have the same effect. Researchers have made recent discoveries, and special attention is being paid to two hormones: leptin and ghrelin.

Leptin was discovered in 1994. It is produced in fat tissues peripherally, but it connects and communicates with the hypothalamus (a part of the brain that regulates appetite, heart rate, blood pressure, sleep, temperature, etc.). Scientists believe it plays a role in signaling the amount of fat to be stored in the body, therefore causing changes in the desire, appetite, and urge for fat consumption based on what is in storage. It is the stop sign on the street corner. This hormone is supposed to tell us this: "You are not hungry anymore. Cease and desist with the eating." Leptin is there to suppress our appetites and helps us burn calories. Each person has a different leptin threshold. When the amount of leptin is low (leptin deficiency) or if it is no longer effective, the body becomes leptin resistant. When this occurs, there is no gatekeeper to regulate and tell when the level of fats is enough and when we are full. Leptin is no longer there to decrease or suppress appetite, which explains why obese people have high levels of leptin but are still obese. Therefore, we do not get the stop signal, and we drive straight ahead having no idea that we are no longer hungry. The deficiency or resistance of leptin causes the person to continue overeating. This could be another explanation for obesity; however, more studies are needed and are currently ongoing.

Ghrelin was discovered in the stomach in 1999. It stimulates appetite. When the stomach is empty, the amount of ghrelin increases considerably, then, through the bloodstream, it crosses the blood-brain barrier and—like leptin—reaches the region of the hypothalamus that deals with food intake to signal hunger. As the stomach receives nutrients, ghrelin no longer sends the "I'm hungry" signal.

Leptin and ghrelin play key roles in regulating our appetites and affecting our weights. While leptin controls our appetites, ghrelin tells us we need more food.

Researchers are working diligently to get a handle on the right balance to keep our weights in check.

There are other hormones that also contribute to the accumulation of body fat, such as insulin resistance in the diabetic as well as sex and growth hormones. Besides affecting our weights, hormonal imbalance can also cause various types of maladies, including prostate, breast, and ovarian cancers; autoimmune diseases; and other medical issues such as diabetes and hypertension. Hormones such as thyroid, insulin, cortisol, estrogens, testosterone, progesterone, etc., not only influence our weights, but they are themselves often affected by other causes. Hormones fluctuate under the influence of the aging process, gender, nutritional habits, level of activity, as well as some environmental factors such as pesticides, herbicides, chemicals, and industrial substances that we use and even ingest in our daily lives.

Furthermore, as if this is not enough, our lifestyles—the level of stress, the number of hours invested in our sleep, and our overall health—also affect our hormonal functions. Hormonal fluctuations and instability should be taken into account especially when we are experiencing symptoms such as malaise, fatigue, general slowness, insomnia, change in appetite and sleep habits, osteoporosis, change in hair and skin texture, mood swings, irritability, infertility, breast enlargement, decrease in muscle mass, difficulty concentrating, impotence, or decrease in libido. Because most people do not really know much about their endocrine functions, it is advised that a hormonal check should be part of any responsible weight-loss plan. In addition, sleep has been found to be very important in obesity prevention. It is thought that having less than six hours of uninterrupted sleep at night is a risk for obesity and other health problems. People who work at night and sleep during the day are also at risk.

## Emotional/Psychological Factors

Because obesity has reached an epidemic proportion, more and more issues related to such a condition are also reported. People who are obese are made self-conscious of their weights by other people's reactions, jokes, and comments. They tend to be stereotyped as lazy and slow, with low self-esteem and lack of willpower and discipline. Because of society's bias and ambivalence toward obese people, they are victims of discrimination in the job market, work environment, schools and general educational settings, and even while seeing their health-care providers. Therefore, it is not surprising that many obese people often feel stigmatized with psychological consequences. They may be bored, depressed, sad, stressed, frustrated, angry, etc. Because food is easily accessible at gas stations, movie theaters, restaurants, supermarkets, airports, and on almost every table in the house, it becomes a simple reflex to turn to eating as a way to cope with these issues. Some people tend to eat even when they are not hungry because they are looking for ways to satisfy some of their inner needs or urges. Eating may become a coping mechanism. Obese people may shy away from physical activities because they are not sure they want to be seen. This pattern of behavior places them in a situation in which the result is the opposite of what they would like to accomplish.

Qualified, professional interventions are required to help those of us who are in such a situation to obtain psychological improvement. These steps may include some positive coping strategies, empathy and support groups to develop self-acceptance, and behavioral modifications for healthy life transformations. In addition, governments need to take measures against all types of discrimination, including against obese and overweight people. (The government also needs to offer incentives or preventive measures against obesity as the burden of obesity is carried by everyone in society in the form of health-care costs and decreased productivity.) After all, we come in different sizes and shapes, but all of us have our place under the sun. The charm of life lies in its varieties.

## Medications

All of us want a healthy and vibrant life. Unfortunately, some of us are either born with illnesses or we develop health conditions that require medical attention. As such, in many instances, we have to take medications that might contribute to becoming overweight or obese. The list of medications that cause such results includes steroids; anticancer medications; nonsteroidal anti-inflammatory drugs (NSAIDs); and medications for depression, migraines, seizures, high-blood pressure, diabetes, and psychiatric conditions. There are instances in which there are no substitutes, no other alternatives. The proper approach is to discuss the issue with a competent doctor or get a second opinion if needed for optimal management of your medical condition. At any rate, do not just stop the medications without consulting and having a clear discussion with your doctor.[7]

---

7 *The Annals of Pharmacotherapy.* Vol. 39, no. 12, pp. 2046–2054. Google: DNA double helix picture doi: 10.1345/aph.1G33.

## Social Factors

Obese people may develop a feeling of inadequacy. They may also be victims of discrimination, thoughtlessness, teasing, and bullying and cruel comments. They may feel lonely or ashamed about their appearances. Unfortunately, instead of turning things around, the obese person may turn to food and may withdraw from his or her peers and fall into a vicious cycle that can only contribute to further weight gain. Sadly, it is a vicious cycle.

## Viruses

Although many of the causes of obesity have been identified, some have not. Scientific research continues to grow and make great gains in this area. By the turn of the twenty-first century, researchers have added other possibilities, including the discovery of a handful of viruses as a possible contributing factor to obesity. They affect the existing fat cells in the body and also recruit, convert, and mature new fat cells to expand fat storage.

## Culture, Ethnicity, and Obesity

Although we are all unique individuals, we cannot easily separate ourselves from the beliefs, values, customs, and behavioral patterns that are part of our common thread and fabric. Yes, we have reached a point where the world is a global village; however, certain characteristics remain typical for each nation, ethnicity, region, and community. In some ways, it is because of this that no culture is immune from obesity. Certain cultural idiosyncrasies may actually encourage obesity!

In some cultures, women who have curves are preferred over those who look thinner. Some cultures have specific unhealthy foods as a part their rituals. It may even be a cultural norm for children to eat everything on their plates, even when they are not hungry or when the portions are too much for them! In some places, a good appetite is a compliment to the chef or the host. There may be a cultural or ethnic reason behind why some people must take and eat as much as they can from a buffet restaurant to make sure they have eaten their money's worth. Cultural competency and even social class influence obesity and weight management.

## Religion

Obviously, in our quest to identify the causes of obesity, no stone must be left unturned. This explains why some people suggest that religion may influence and sometimes even encourage obesity. In some religious gatherings, it is not farfetched to wonder how certain habits may have an influence on obesity. When people gather to pray, praise, and worship, they also tend to eat together as part of their fellowship. Potlucks are common in many churches. However, the drive to prepare the best dish at the potluck may not give rise to the healthiest ones. The results are often high-calorie, unhealthy meals. For example, I cannot recall if I have ever been to a church potluck that did not have tasty fried foods.

However, the time has come to review the meaning of eating well to make sure it also means eating healthy. So the greasy, salty, sugary meals, the cookies, candies, cakes, and ice cream should be examined along with the portion size! We must be conscious of what we are serving to others. The time has come to review dietary habits at church gatherings as well as individual church members' eating habits. How can we change what may be a tradition without people becoming defensive?

## National Policies and Dietary Guidelines

Our awareness about the increasing percentage of people who have become overweight and obese must lead us to review the global and national politics and policies that affect our weights. We have allowed unhealthy foods to rein almost everywhere, beginning in schools, although some school districts have started to ban sugary drinks from vending machines and to serve more healthful school meals in response to the childhood obesity epidemic. People are bombarded with advertising for junk food and high-calorie drinks rich in sugar. Conflicts often arise between the government and the general public on one side and the powerful food industry on the other. The food industry pursues one goal, which is of course to continue to make a profit. Until there is a consensus to implement policies, dietary guidelines, and environmental strategies that foster healthier nutritional choices and a change in priorities, the fight against obesity will remain just a bunch of empty rhetoric. Obesity is not a Republican, Democrat, or Independent issue. It concerns all of us on the planet. Two monumental changes that have come about in recent years are the trans-fat ban and the requirement for chain restaurants to label calories—both required the government to step up. Instead of providing government subsidies to the corn, wheat, beef, milk, and soybean industries, government could perhaps subsidize fruits and vegetables to make them more affordable. Another discussion has been to prevent people who receive food stamps (SNAP) from buying sugary drinks and unhealthful foods, but this is proving highly controversial.

The treatment for obesity must not raise only a global concern, but it also requires a conjugated effort from all sectors to reverse the trend and bring about a durable and effective solution. It cannot be solely a private, individual matter but instead a comprehensive, well-grounded, integrated, multidisciplinary strategy. Some may argue that obesity should be treated as smoking was treated—a societal health risk requiring the government to intervene.

The most challenging time to keep the weight under control includes infancy, adolescence, during and post pregnancy, and around menopause.

Overall, obesity is a disease with many causes and consequences. Some of these causes include ignoring our bodies' hunger/satiety cues, ages and genders, the types of food available and consumed, lack of exercise, high levels of stress, rates of metabolism, genetics, DNA methylation, lack of sleep, environments, biochemistry, metabolic abnormalities, behavioral conditions, social networks, viruses, intestinal microflora, hormonal fluctuations, cultural norms, and certain medical conditions. As more research is performed, we may encounter other contributing factors to obesity.

## Different People, Different Factors

Another way of putting it is that obesity is due to different factors for different people. The key is for researchers to continue with studies and findings to shed light on the various causes of obesity and for everyone to take steps to identify the reasons for their individual conditions and address them to the best of their abilities.

# CHAPTER 4

## Consequences of Being Obese

Because of obesity, there is an increase in the likelihood of developing various medical conditions and health risks. Obesity can greatly influence lifestyle, and in fact, in can cause secondary medical conditions and eventually premature death. Following are a few examples of conditions associated with or caused by obesity.

### On Physical Illness

As part of the consequences of obesity, here is a list of medical burdens that can occur:

- High blood pressure
- Diabetes mellitus (DM)
- Metabolic syndrome—a condition in which a person has three of the following: large waist circumference,

high level of sugar in the blood, high blood pressure, low good cholesterol (HDL), or high triglycerides
- Fatty liver
- Atherosclerosis (fatty deposits obstructing the walls of the arteries)
- Headaches/migraines
- Coronary heart disease
- Respiratory difficulty/pulmonary dysfunction
- Sleep apnea (when breathing stops on and off during sleep, which can be dangerous)
- Sluggishness
- Blood clots or venous stasis/insufficiency
- Stroke
- Gout
- Gallbladder disease and gallstones
- Arthritis/joint pain or cramps
- Malaise and fatigue
- Impaired mobility
- Back pain
- Difficulty breathing/asthma
- Heartburn or gastro esophageal reflux disease
- High cholesterol and triglycerides
- Hormonal imbalance
- Hernia
- Erectile dysfunction
- Cellulitis

- Delayed wound healing
- Carpal tunnel syndrome
- Urinary incontinence
- Infertility/subfertility or menstrual irregularities
- Constipation
- Hearing impairment
- Polycystic ovarian syndrome
- Renal insufficiency/failures
- Certain types of cancer

These medical conditions do not share an identical pre-dominance. However, not only do they affect the quality of life of overweight people but also their surroundings and their caretakers. Some of these even cause disability and premature death!

## On Mental Health

Although the physical signs of obesity are obvious, the psychological and emotional effects are no less important. Those who do not fit the standard mold of what is acceptable in appearance internalize a number of psychological scars. Obesity may hamper familial stability, and even limit professional success. It may provide an excuse for subtle discrimination, and affect even one's salary and promotion. Obesity may also have an impact on general feelings or mood. It may cause malaise, fatigue, feeling sluggish, and depression. It may also encourage poor self-image, anxiety, or the progression of eating disorders. Other factors related to mental health are social stigmatization, sexual dissatisfaction, poverty and ultimately premature mortality.

## Other Suggested Factors Related to Obesity

It is interesting to note that in Greek comedy, a fat character, Obesus, was seen as someone who was silly, and in Charles Dickens's nineteenth-century novel *The Pickwick Papers*, obese people were caricaturized. Obese people were perceived as weak willed, gluttonous, lazy, depressed, ugly, and the subject of mockery. It was a cause for discrimination. In a few instances, obesity may have generated racial, social, and familial sneers and insults. In this example, we see how obesity can be mocked and influence one's life.

When dealing with the issue of obesity, we are not merely dealing with "being fat"; the challenge has to do with how other people may perceive us. The ideas about obesity—that obese people eat too much; lack self-control; are lazy, unhealthy, and overindulgent; or are devoid of romantic relationships with emotional issues—are still not completely eradicated. In fact, they may even be perpetuated by the media. Let us, for example, take the movie *The Nutty Professor*—the entire Klump family is a cause for ridicule, and the main character is a professor! You may say it is a comedy, so it is supposed to be funny. Think hard. When is the last time you saw an overweight character starring in a show that was not a comedy? The list of TV shows and movies that have overweight stars includes *The Parkers*, *The Office*, *Family Guy*, *Paul Blart: Mall Cop*, and *Fat Albert*. I am hard pressed to find a show in which the fat character is taken seriously. How many shows would go out featuring slim, healthy, and sexy people in a comedy?

Notwithstanding, obesity decreases life expectancy, increases health-care costs, and decreases work productivity. To put it forthrightly, obesity should be a matter of national security. It is not only a matter of life and death but affects daily life as well. Every person who is overweight or obese is different and has unique issues that require special attention and care. However, we are in dire need of a way to address it individually and globally, considering the high rate of diseases resulting from obesity and the health and social consequences that have followed.

# CHAPTER 5

## Eleven Myths Regarding Overweight and Obesity

*M*yth 1: *All calories are the same.* Nothing is further from the truth. From a metabolic perspective, not all calories are created equal. It has to do with the source of the caloric intake. The term *empty calories* refers to foods that are often high in calories yet offer no nutritional benefits—for example, candies and sugar-sweetened beverages. In addition, the effect of those empty calories items depends on whether the calories come from processed or whole, basic foods.

*Myth 2: To stay healthy and fit, you cannot have any fun.* Nowhere is it stated that you need to have an austere and misanthropic life. It is impossible to have rigid dietary guidelines and never, ever stray. To quote Alexander Pope, "To err is human." We know that staying healthy and fit requires a decision to change behavior and to divorce from the old ways of doing things. We need to adopt a practical, livable, balanced diet that is appropriate for each one of us. Deprivation is not what we should be aiming for. If you want to have a piece of fried chicken once in a while at a church potluck or a special occasion, go for it, as long as you are not going to make it a permanent lifestyle. Remember, the goal is to keep the pounds off.

*Myth 3: Dieting is for a few days or before a special occasion.* That may be true for dieting, but we are aiming for a truly lifetime endeavor in which we consider the quantity and quality of our food intake on a daily basis. Yes, that sounds tedious. However, after a few days doing it, it will become second nature. We will automatically know when our portions are too big. This is merely to encourage us to take the proper steps to help us succeed. As important as portion size is choosing the right foods and keeping the undesirable foods out of the house.

It is a new lifestyle. It is also a new state of mind that we have decided to take on. Therefore, we cannot approach it with a long face as if it were a punishment, a purge, or some sort of bitter medicine to be tolerated for a few days. No! Instead, let us take the steps to make it as enjoyable as possible. If we begrudge the process before we even begin, we will not continue to do it daily.

*Myth 4: Those who follow a particular regime are malnourished or have some deficiencies.* Many people think that adopting a diet different from the one they have been used to their entire lives can cause problems or make them sick. In reality, adopting a balanced diet in which the proportions of macronutrients and micronutrients are right improves health. Avoid a rapid decline in weight caused by starvation. Weight that is lost through deprivation will usually not stay off! Remember that your food needs to change as you move through the cycle of life and when you move to a different country or environment.

*Myth 5: The idea of a healthy diet suggests a bland, limited, and boring menu day in and day out.* It is a lie! It is important to understand the meaning of the word *diet*. It only means reducing the amount of calories/energy intake by decreasing the overall food intake or increasing your calories expenditures. There are many healthy dishes that are delicious and that you will enjoy eating. Some are even easy to prepare. The key is to vary the menu and adapt the food of your culture. For this, there are many resources available, including searching the Internet with discernment. A daily meal choice can be found by using Google or other apps. Nowadays, we have a wealth of information at our fingertips and many ways in which we can vary our diets.

*Myth 6: Most people often go back to or even beyond their initial weights because they cannot keep healthy habits.* I am sure many of you can provide anecdotal evidence to prove this true. We could probably discuss this for hours. However, the fact is, after losing a certain number of pounds, it becomes more and more difficult to keep it up because our bodies and our rates of metabolism learn to adjust to the new weights. We need fewer calories to function at our new level of body mass. Our human tendency is to measure results based on the number reflected on the scale. That is not accurate. Sometimes we may lose on size, inches, and fat, while our bodies become firmer and more muscular. The main idea is not to be so obsessed about the whole process but to keep track of our daily activities, diets, and all other factors that can affect our healthy lifestyles. Then, let the rest take care of itself.

*Myth 7: The pounds lost are directly proportional to how much we eat and how active we are.* That is not usually so! This is not the hard-and-fast rule! The causes of obesity are multifactorial, and everyone is different. The right approach is to find the weight, the contour, and the shape we are comfortable with. We cannot measure our success according to others' performances. Every one of us is a unique being, and the factors and results differ accordingly. Furthermore, weight loss alone may not provide the ideal result. Our genetic predispositions and other factors must also be taken into account.

*Myth 8: Eating between meals increases the chance of obesity.* Before you jump up and down, let me explain. Logically, this sounds right. However, the fact is that on your whole daily menu, snacking is not the problem. As a matter of fact, besides the three regular meals, snacking is highly recommended, but not if it drastically increases daily intake. The key is what kinds of snack we take in. We should stay away from candies, cookies, popcorn, crackers and cheese, and simple carbohydrates rich in sugars, calories and fats. Instead, we should choose whole foods such as fruits; plain, low-fat yogurt; and a small portion of nuts, some dried fruit, and raw vegetables.

The key concept here is to read the label on what looks like a harmless, quick snack and judge if you really, really want it after all the progress you have made. Sometimes that box of Oreos may just not be worth it—or maybe one Oreo, depending on your emotional or physical state.

*Myth 9: A good diet means changing your entire food intake into low fat.* WHAT? Although many people used to believe this, it is no longer a widely held belief. The expression *low fat* can be misleading if it gives us the impression that it will keep our body fat low—quite the contrary: eating some of the right kind of fat makes us feel full and satisfied on less food. Rather than focusing on "low fat" or "low calorie," focusing on the types of foods we put into our bodies is more important. As previously mentioned, to overcome obesity, it is necessary to adopt a lifestyle change rather than just dieting. Diets often cannot be followed over the course of a lifetime, whereas behavioral changes can be. We must also take into account certain medical conditions. For example, if a diabetic patient has to choose between an apple and a banana, both fruits may be good in and of themselves, but the sugar content in a banana is somewhat higher than in the apple. This would make the apple the better choice based on that individual's condition. But if the patient liked bananas, I would prefer that they eat the fresh fruit.

*Myth 10: To lose weight, we must stay away from carbohydrates.* With the advent of a ton of diets that encourage low or no carbs, we can easily interpret carbs as "making us fat."

Nothing is further from the truth. To stay healthy, a well-balanced diet is necessary to provide enough calories for the body to function properly. This includes protein, fat, and carbohydrates with essential nutrients, fiber, vitamins, and minerals. Carbohydrates play an important role as our first source of energy and a source of vital vitamins and minerals. The difference is in the type of carbohydrate that is consumed. As a matter of fact, more than 50 percent of our caloric intake is provided by complex carbohydrates.

What we need to do is avoid simple/refined carbohydrates, which are found in candies, cookies, or sugar-sweetened beverages that are high in calories, low in nutrients, and high in refined sugars, causing the pancreas to release more and more insulin, which in turn promotes the storage of excess energy as fat. Of course, we should eat carbohydrates, but they should be complex carbohydrates such as those found in fruits, vegetables, and brown rice and whole grains.

*Myth 11: I was born to be obese; nothing can change that.* There is clear evidence that some people are more prone to obesity than others. There is also evidence that these people can make changes in their lives to change their conditions. These changes include the types of foods they eat, portion sizes, levels of physical activity and motivation, and daily habits. These steps and others do make a difference in people's health. So, do not, under any circumstances, give up hope. In persevering, many people have changed their "fates."

In conclusion, we must realize the obesity epidemic does indeed affect us all. We need appropriate knowledge and to be apprised of scientific fact to be better equipped to have a handle on it. Here are a few basic facts we must remember:

1. We know we need carbohydrates as a main source of energy, but the secret is in the choices we make

regarding the quality and the quantity we take in. We must go for whole foods such as the following:

a. fruits—apples, blueberries, kiwis, strawberries, oranges, bananas, papaya, and grapes

b. vegetables—broccoli, cauliflower, asparagus, sweet potatoes, carrots, cabbage, spinach, leafy greens, and low-sodium vegetable juices

c. legumes—beans, including pinto, kidney, black, red, lentils, chickpeas, and green peas

d. whole grains—oatmeal, brown rice, wild rice, barley, buckwheat, whole grain or wheat bread, wild rice, and millet

2. We need protein for muscle build up and repair. However, we must be careful in our source of proteins. Good sources include wild salmon or any other oily fish such as blue fish, herring, mackerel, and sardines; tuna; white-meat poultry; organic eggs; yogurt; beans; and soy products.

3. We need fat to cushion our organs, protect our joints, and help our bodies absorb necessary nutrients. The difference is in our source of fat. Fats should be unsaturated; sources include fish (salmon, mackerel, sardines, tuna, and herring), olive and sunflower oil, avocados, olives (these can be high in sodium), and nuts and seeds. Some saturated animal fats can be part of balanced meals,

especially small servings of organic, grass-fed beef and low-fat milk and real cheese.

While doing all of the above, we should avoid going through the same routine daily or eating foods like white flours, sweets, and refined and highly processed products. These are treats! Choosing unfavorable foods daily will affect our metabolisms and weights and cause bloating, malaise, fatigue, and abdominal pain as well as affect our moods and our interactions with others.

# CHAPTER 6

## The Peculiarity of Obesity

Food intake has always played an important role for people throughout the ages. All the special gatherings since the genesis of the world have usually revolved around eating, drinking, and having fun. However, not everybody becomes obese. In fact, until recently, it was a tiny minority. What has changed? One cannot zero in only on food. There must be other factors. Regarding our diets, we must question what has changed in our environments, our daily activities, our eating habits, and the type, quality, and quantity of foods we eat to cause such drastic consequences.

With the advent of globalization, the effect of instant communication is that the pattern of occidentalization is flourishing. The Western hemisphere sets the tone. It has glorified fast, junk, processed foods with a lot of fat and sugar. They taste good and are less expensive than "yucky" fruits and vegetables. With the advent of the fast-food industry and food advertising, the Western world has exported its habits and even imposed its ever-changing cultures on the rest of the world. Obesity has become prevalent in the current population worldwide and is on the rise in developing countries.

Shortly after some people began to consume and condone "junk food", they started to notice its effects. In addition, because now we are calling attention to the ever-increasing percentage of people who will become obese, especially among children, the whole world is reacting to what Dr. Sander Gilman called *"globesity*.[8]

Toward the end of the twentieth century, the WHO declared obesity to be a global epidemic.[9] The United States has unfortunately made the list of top-twenty most-obese countries in the world. As a worldwide issue, every nation is concerned about it and wants to come up with a lasting solution.

Nevertheless, this does not prevent some people from doubting whether obesity is such a life-threatening issue, at least of the magnitude that is publicized worldwide. In reality, some may say, it is not even among the top causes

8  Gilman, Sander L., Obesity: The Biography (Biographies of Disease) 1st Edition, Oxford University Press

9  Bhurosy, Trishnee and Rajesh Jeewon, The Scientific World Journal, Volume 2014 (2014), Article ID 964236, 7 pages http://dx.doi.org/10.1155/2014/964236, Review Article www.who.int/dietphysicalactivity/media/en/gsfs_obesity.

of death in the United States or worldwide. Nevertheless, obesity contributes to major causes of death in many cases, including heart disease, diabetes, and cancer.

## The Advantages of Obesity

This heading may come as a surprise for many. It is not very often that we think of the "advantages" of being overweight. Nevertheless, we need to bear in mind that we are not born with the same height, weight, size, and shape as everyone else. There are families in which all members are genetically predisposed to have bigger builds with larger bones. These people distinguish themselves by being perfect in their own skin and should aspire only to be their healthiest and not as skinny as some celebrities. If they are active and follow a healthy lifestyle, that should be conducive to good health. Perhaps you are the only one who can lift that bag of goods after a day of shopping with friends. Perhaps your strong bones provide you with the means to do things your "skinny-minny" friends cannot even fathom attempting. As a matter of fact, you may even enjoy being huge, imposing, and intimidating. That may give you the advantage of being left alone when a circumstance would warrant a fight. In many cases, a man's physical appearance may keep him from the threat of violence.

Furthermore, researchers have reported instances in which obesity may produce a protective effect against future heart conditions for people who have had heart disease. This is called the "obesity paradox." Further investigations are ongoing. But it could be because the body of an obese person has endured so much that after a heart attack, the increased health awareness that forces a better lifestyle is good enough to have a protective effect. However, it is still recommended that we maintain a weight in a healthy range to prevent the development of certain chronic conditions in the first place.

Another advantage that obese people might have is acting in specific roles. Think of *The Sopranos* character Dominic "Fat Dom" Gamiello. Would it really have been the same if he were skinny?

Overall, regardless of our size, the key is to be fully functional and to lower the chances of becoming sick or disabled or dying prematurely from obesity-related causes. Those of us who happen to be born with predisposition to be on the heavy side can still benefit from staying fit and keeping healthy habits. At times, environment can overcome our genetic predispositions.

In addition, as we age and get older and older, weight will definitely make a difference in our health and fitness. Some in the health discipline believe that being slightly overweight may be beneficial for older people (with a BMI up to twenty-nine). But for younger people, anything we do to lose weight, fortify our bones and muscles, stay agile, and take care of our daily activities is commendable and worthy of praise and encouragement. It is beneficial to our health and well-being. It prepares us for later days when we may not be able to follow the strict diet recommended.

Although there are a lot of alarming media reports about obesity and its morbidity and mortality, some countries, including the United States, have not yet seen the full effect or severity of obesity, such as the increased health-care costs for people with long-term conditions like type 2 diabetes. Many wonder if the broad desire for globalization—to have one huge economy, one huge culture, one huge political system—is being represented—even subconsciously—as a desire to have uniformity in people's sizes, heights, weights. How much do politics, media, and global hysteria play into the big commotion about obesity?

Unfortunately, only time will tell. However, it is official that obesity in itself is a disease. We cannot stay passive and ignore its secondary and tertiary effects on the nation's and world's population.

# CHAPTER 7

## Why Is Obesity So Prevalent?

The increased availability of the "wrong" types of food that are easily accessible strongly urges us to eat even when we are not hungry. We have come to ignore our hunger and satiety cues that the body gives. In times before, fruits, legumes, vegetables, fish, and meat had to be gathered and prepared at home. Families used to gather and eat just what they needed for healthy meals. There was no such thing as surplus, and families included grandparents and other extended family as well, which is not so today.

With the advent of technology, economic strain, and changes in sociocultural structures, a change was made to coincide with lifestyle changes. Most of us have to work long hours, so of course there is no time to cook. Instead, we grasp onto whatever comes our way in and out of work or home, mainly fast-food restaurants and junk food. Do not get me wrong; sometimes these foods come to our "rescue" and are the only recourse. However, then we develop a dependency on them. We develop a habit of munching on potato chips day in and day out. Perhaps we grow a little health conscious and grab some baked or "natural" chips. It is convenient. However, these types of choices call for an increased consumption of sugar, salt, and saturated fat. It feels like we are always pressed for time, so we sacrifice healthy, nutritious foods. There does not seem to be time to exchange grandma's recipes anymore. Everything is premade, ready to eat, or microwaveable. Before the Industrial Revolution, our food-supply chain was very different. Meat was more expensive as the amount of resources required to grow a calf into a cow is vastly greater than growing vegetables. It has become much easier to produce meat in large quantities due to the industrialization of the food supply. This change in our food-supply chain has largely affected the composition of our diets worldwide—no longer is meat the food of the rich. Likewise, we are starting to see diseases of the "rich man" such as gout and obesity become more prevalent in the general population.

It has gotten so bad that our children's taste buds are so used to junk food that the only time they eat an apple is when they are sliced and prepackaged and sold at Subway. It has become a reward for good behavior to take children to a fast-food restaurant. There is almost no room for fresh fruits, legumes, salads, and vegetables. Youngsters judge essential nutrients as bland, boring, and old-fashioned. Furthermore, there is even less time for outdoor walks or trips to the playground or any other form of physical activity. Besides, the situation is even more nuanced because of the potential for criminality that children may face in public parks.

Simply put, some of us just have a great appetite for unhealthy food. We take large portions of food and resolve in our hearts to clean our plates. We may even eat more than we need and more often than we should. For example, people who attend more than one Christmas dinner will seldom refuse a plate. They feel obligated to indulge in multiple meals to appear gracious to their hosts, even though they know they are beyond full. Interestingly, the larger the plate, the more food will be eaten—restaurants (and people) have increased their plate sizes! Hence, more food on the plate.

Furthermore, we tend not to pay attention to the content of what we ingest. "Bad" foods (rich in empty calories, poor in nutrients, and high in fat, salt, sugar, and chemicals) are easily accessible and considerably cheap. They taste great and look appealing even when our stomachs are full. For example, Kool-Aid is very affordable. It contains ascorbic acid (Vitamin C—a better source is a fruit), several chemicals, artificial colors, maltodextrin (a type of sugar), and salt, and some flavors have added sugar. Nevertheless, it tastes so good! A regular can of soda is just carbonated water, sweetener, and chemicals. I am not saying that you should give up Kool-Aid or soda! I am merely suggesting that you choose water more often. It is interesting to note that usually when we are craving sweets or a sweet beverage, it really means we are thirsty. Next time you have that feeling, try drinking a glass of water before reaching for what you are craving.

Some people use overeating as a way to cope with stress, frustration, and depression. Food gives them a sense of belonging, acceptance, and importance. For these people, I would suggest learning new coping skills. Instead of grabbing that cupcake, perhaps a lavender-scented bath might ease your pain. Or meditation, prayer, or yoga might do the trick.

For some people, eating out is their only source of pleasure and self-actualization. Regardless of how and where they get the food, once they get to eat, they feel licensed to order absolutely anything because the only thing that pleases them is eating. Perhaps reading this book and kick starting an active life will not be enough for these people. I would encourage them to consult a doctor and share their concerns. A trip to Overeaters Anonymous would also not be a bad idea. Do not be ashamed. Do not give up. You may just need a little extra support to get well.

People may gain weight because of additives in our foods that make us feel good. Popular foods often taste great and flatter our taste buds. We have become used to a diet filled with a lot of sugar, salt, spices, and gravy. In addition, we also become obese because of secondary effects: the poor quality of foods (toxicity, pathogens, and infections), certain chemicals like MSG (monosodium glutamate) added to the food to make it tastier, preservatives, food coloring, sugar consumption, and toxins.

There has also been a change in work environments. Technology has made transportation less physical. There is an increase in amusements such as television, the Internet, video games, social media, and smartphones. People no longer have to get up and go to the computer to send an e-mail; they can send you a four-paragraph missive from their beds. Our workforce is more service oriented with less physically demanding labor and decreased walking. These factors have made it much easier for us to gain weight.

## Analysis of the Situation

Obviously, there is a worldwide increase in obesity. Many more people are becoming aware of this condition. However, there is no consensus when it comes to the clear and definite causes and the treatment of obesity. There are people who eat a lot who are still slim and fit, while others seem to just smell the food and gain weight. This is why research is being pursued to find a definitive formula to address obesity in various people living in the same environmental conditions with different results.

There have been a few leads in research, including the discovery of genetic predisposition. Various other leads are being followed up to come up with a solution. It is clear that the correct approach is to consider several factors, including identifying all the biomarkers, categorizing them, and classifying people based on their specific biomarkers; the role of the brain (hypothalamus); neuroendocrine system; psychosocial factors; the environment; politics; public policy; public relations; and education. All of these and many more factors need to be addressed to find the right solution to this growing problem.

So far, the solutions proposed are better nutrition, stress management, paired coaching, increased education, more exercise, portion control, behavior modification, mindful eating, healthy eating, meal planning, public policy, and avoidance of certain foods. All these steps have their roles, but they do not seem to fix the problem completely.

Many people are willing to go on a diet and to exercise. However, not many are willing to change their lifestyles. Many reach a plateau, which seems to be impassable, and they do not seem to be able to lose any more weight and give up altogether. After some time, the body becomes more efficient and adjusts to the weight decrease by using less energy at rest or during activities; it decides to store a bit more of each meal, preparing for what might be a famine. This is why, after a while, it becomes necessary to use other aids and make adjustments to reach your ideal weight.

Let us revisit the factors that determine our weights:

1. *Genetic inheritance:* This is the package inherited from our parents and what we come into the world with.
2. *Basal metabolic rate:* This is based on height, weight, age, gender, health condition, and body composition; we have a set number of calories that are needed to keep us going daily. If we get more calories than we need, the excess is stored as fat. If we use more calories than we eat in foods, we lose weight. If we get as many calories as we spend, then weight is maintained.
3. *Eating habits:* This has to do with the quality and quantity of our nutrition.
4. *Level of activity:* This refers to both exercise in itself and our overall daily ability to move and use our muscles.
5. *Lifestyle:* This includes mealtimes, length and quality of sleep, and day or night work. Wait a minute! This is <u>not</u> as simple as it sounds. When we start

losing weight, after a while, the body adjusts to our new eating habits. If it realizes that you are eating less, than it starts becoming more energy efficient both at rest and during activities because it is programmed to deal better with starvation than overabundance. This is why you should not go on a crash diet for a few days because the effects will not last. You must not starve yourself or go on a restrictive diet for any reason. Your eating habits should be plugged on a lasting curve by watching what you eat and how much you eat and becoming more conscious of what you put in your body.

# PART II
## How to Face the Challenge of Obesity

# CHAPTER 8

## Deciphering the Yo-Yo Phenomenon of Weight Loss and Gain

Anna is in her late twenties; she is five foot seven and weighs 150 pounds. Bill is in his early thirties; he is five foot four and weighs 150 pounds. They are both well acquainted with current events, and both know that health care is a hotly debated issue. They would like to take steps not only to be part of the long life forecasted for younger generations but also would like to stay healthy and fit. What are the comprehensive steps they can take to reach such a goal?

**Step 1:** The idea of weight control requires that each of us knows our current weights, the number of calories we consume every day, and our levels of activity. This means you are able to answer the following:

1. What is your age, gender, height, health status, and weight?

2. How many calories do you use on a daily basis? How much do you eat? How many calories are necessary for your level of functioning? Here are some specifics: depending on their activity, a man needs an average of 2,000–2,500 calories daily; a woman needs an average of 1,500–2,000 calories daily. If we are among those who consume much more than these amounts, then the challenge is to meet the minimum required to make a significant difference in our weights. But the harder the task, the greater the satisfaction when it is accomplished. However, we must be careful not to put ourselves into starvation mode as weight loss then becomes almost impossible. In other words, there is a minimum of intake calories needed for everyone.[10]

3. What is your usual activity level? Are you sedentary, lightly active, moderately active, or athletic? Do you do strenuous work (construction)? Your physical activity level will influence your estimated energy needs.

---

10 **US Department of Agriculture. https://www.cnpp.usda.gov/USDAFood-Patterns**

**Step 2**: The next step on our weight-management journey is to be diligent. To prove our commitment, we must acquire as much knowledge as possible while filtering out ideas that circulate but are not supported scientifically. Anna and Bill need to be familiar with certain concepts such as BMI, body mass ratio, and the height and weight chart.

To make it more practical, let us take the raw data submitted by Anna and Bill. Based on what is already known, the two must establish whether their weights are normal, below normal, or above normal. To do so, they need to look at the height and weight chart, which classifies weight according to height and gender. It is there they will discover what the ideal weight for Anna is, as well as the ideal weight for Bill. Then, they will be able to determine whether or not they are over the mark, even if it is not by much, and what to do about it.

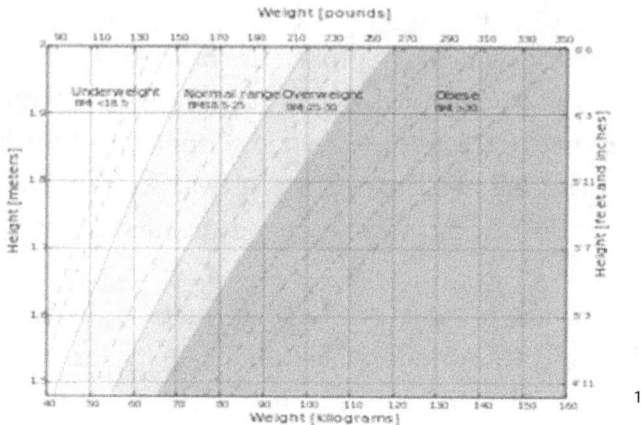

According to common BMI charts, including one provided by www.disabled-world.com, Vertex42.com, or Wikipedia (above), they can see what is the number they pivot around. If Anna and Bill are conscious about their weights now and take action, they can keep them under control, improve their muscle tone, and even circumvent some health conditions that may be genetic or environmental without risky dieting. However, if they realize they are somehow over the mark, if they fail to do anything about it, there is a chance they will accumulate more weight due to the aging process (which slows metabolism), environmental factors, and lifestyle. If the trend continues, they may even become obese. (By the way,

---

11 wikipedia.org/wiki/Body_mass_index.

there are apps for our smartphone that can calculate BMI, ideal weight, etc., to help us stay on track.)

### BMI Weight Status Categories

| BMI | Weight Status |
| --- | --- |
| Below 18.5 | Underweight |
| 18.5–24.9 | Normal |
| 25.0–29.9 | Overweight |
| 30.0 and above | Obese |
| 40.0 and above | Morbidly Obese |

**Step 3**: Once we have discovered where we are regarding our current weights and ideal weights, regardless of the numbers, the next step is not to be complacent if you fall within the normal range and not to panic if you do not. Instead, you need to be proactive and decide to get in shape and stay in shape.

The key is to set realistic goals. If I am three hundred pounds, my goal cannot be to become a runway model by summer. That is totally pie in the sky. We can have an ultimate big goal, but depending on the individual's age, gender, and rate of metabolism, each step forward may look different. It may take more time than anticipated. It is worth starting slow and building up. A goal set too high will bring discouragement when we fall short of reaching it. So we need to set realistic goals. However, do not decide to abandon your goals—nonchalance and a cavalier attitude will also not serve us. We must have a specific starting and reachable point.

Note that this is not a competition. We do not compete with anyone because everyone is unique. We are not on *The Biggest Loser* television show. Most experts agree that the safe way is to expect <u>to lose one to two pounds per week (0.5–1 kg)</u>. If you eat satisfying whole foods and exercise more, you should be able to achieve such a goal. If you fall short one day, do not be discouraged; the next day you can make up for it if you stay focused. For example, a young lady around her period may not lose any pounds and may even gain some. She may become discouraged and want to quit. After her period, she may find herself sliding back into old habits. She must not lose her focus! We must focus on the big picture and work our way toward reaching the ultimate goal.

**Step 4**: How do we lose one to two pounds a week?

Regardless of the number of pounds we want to lose, we all must begin with basic information as to the mechanism that can help us lose those pounds. Losing weight is not an easy task. As a matter of fact, if we just resume our position as couch potatoes, eating everything within reach, we will most likely gain weight day in and day out, along with all the health issues that come with it.

Yes, losing weight is hard work. Nevertheless, we can do it! This may sound like the cheerleading squad of a losing team chanting out false promises, but it is not. We can accomplish a goal of one or two pounds a week! One of the facts we need to remember is that to lose weight, we must be in an energy deficit each week (spending more energy than we gain). The choice we have is what we eat and how active we become. Ideally, a combination of both is recommended for great success.

1. According to experts, an adult should consume an average of 2,000 calories a day, adolescent 1,250, and child 1,000. How did we arrive at these numbers? The values are not written in stone; they are guides. To be more precise, the first step is to do like Anna and Bill above and reference a height and weight chart. There, based on your gender, height, and weight, you can determine what your ideal weight is. Then you can compare it to your current weight on a reliable scale. If you are like many of us, you will find yourself falling either in the overweight or obese categories. Therefore, the difference between what your actual weight is and your ideal weight should be is the number of extra pounds you have to get rid of, theoretically.

2. When you take that actual weight and use the BMI formula, you can determine if you are over-weight (BMI between twenty-five and thirty) or obese (BMI above thirty).

Although everyone is different, as a general rule, researchers submit three key factors that are involved in determining the total number of daily calories used.

1. **Basal metabolic rate:** Whether we are active or not, it is good to know that our bodies are built to burn two-thirds of caloric intake as a source of energy for our bodies at rest to sustain our heart rates, respiration, sleep, and body temperatures. This is called basal metabolic rate (BMR). BMR is estimated to be equal to the total number of pounds in your body multiplied by ten. For example, if you weigh 150 pounds, your BMR is 1,500 calories (150 × 10). In healthy people, BMR varies with gender (higher in men than women), muscle mass (muscle burns more energy), outside temperature, and hormones, Also, as we age, our BMRs slow down. We tend to store more fat, and metabolism keeps getting slower and slower. One reason is that people tend to eat the same amount when they get older as they did when they were

young! In addition, older people lose muscle mass unless they exercise. To increase BMR, you can build muscle by strength training, increase aerobic exercise (walking or jogging, for example), drink more water, and burn more calories than you consume by eating small meals three to four hours apart. This will cause your BMR to increase because there are fewer calories available at each meal—it works faster to adjust. Otherwise, the more calories it finds available, the more it takes, and its rate decreases.

2. **Physical activity calories:** This has to do with how many calories you burn during your physical activity, which means any movement of your body, not only "exercise." It is calculated by multiplying the BMR by a factor that represents the individual activity level that is a percentage of BMR. This can be anything from the BMR multiplied by 20 percent for an average sedentary lifestyle to the BMR multiplied by 50 percent for an active lifestyle. For example, the physical activity calories for someone with a sedentary lifestyle from the example above is 1,500 × 0.20 = 300 calories, then 300 + 1,500 = 1,800 calories. So 1,800 calories would be that person's total daily allowance. This is the easiest factor to change.

3. **Thermic effect of food:** This concept addresses the number of calories used to digest the foods we ingest. Generally, the digestion factor is calculated to be 10 percent of the total of BMR added to the physical activity calories. In other words, the thermic effect of food or digestion calories from the example above is $1,800 \times 0.10 = 180$ calories. However, it has been found the thermic effect of food may not be a fixed amount, but it may change depending on the type of food we eat. It may be higher if a diet of whole, intact foods (e.g., regular food, home cooked from scratch) is eaten than a diet high in processed foods (e.g., packaged, precooked foods). The body has to work harder and use more energy to digest regular foods than processed foods and snacks.

All in all, for the person in the example to carry out a normal life, he or she must have a total daily caloric expenditure of 1,980 calories (1,500 + 300 + 180).

Let us go back to our example of Anna. She is a five-foot-seven woman who weighs 150 pounds. She wants to reach her ideal weight of 143 pounds. She knows she is seven pounds overweight, and she needs to get rid of the extra weight at a rate of one to two pounds a week. It will take her five to eight weeks without putting her health at risk. Bill is a five-foot-four man who weighs 150 pounds with a target weight of 142 pounds (note that he is a male and is shorter than Anna); he needs to lose eight pounds. He too needs five to eight weeks to get rid of them. Please note, they can also choose to stay at their current weights. It is their choice. No one is forcing us to lose the weight! People can give us advice or encourage us. Nevertheless, it is our lives. We get to make our own decisions.

Both Anna and Bill also must take into account the fact that to lose one pound of fat, they need to burn more calories than are being taken in. How much depends on the person. The saying is to lose one pound of fat per week, you must reduce considerably the number of calories consumed, which can only be a guide and will not work every week, or the same way for everyone. Therefore, to lose one pound of fat a week, each needs to consume about 400 to 500 fewer calories a day (or expend) for the next five to eight weeks. Going from the above calculation, he or she has been consuming 1,980 calories daily. Therefore, he or she needs to subtract 400 to 500 calories from the 1,980 calories. To make the calculation easier with a simpler number, let us state that he or she needs to consume 480 fewer calories daily. So 1,980 - 480 = 1,500 calories; Bill's and Anna's new daily caloric expenditure is 1,500 calories. Therefore, when they spend more calories than they consume, there is a move toward weight loss and vice versa. When they become or remain moderately active and add exercise as part of their daily routines, with all other factors being equal, they will definitely lose the extra weight and stay fit.

Now Anna and Bill need to decide what kinds of food to eat to stay within their 1,500-calorie diets and have their bodies function as usual. Or they could burn 200 calories in exercise and physical activity and decrease their intake by only 300 calories. The best option would be to try eating a 1,500-calorie diet while exercising and being lightly or moderately active. Food modification and reduction work together with exercise for weight loss. This way, Anna and Bill increase the chance of losing even more than what is expected while avoiding starvation mode. Remember, as our journeys to good health continue, there will be good weeks and bad weeks. But it is worth pursuing diligently. The gains are significant.

The ideal choice is to eat more nutrient-dense versus energy-dense foods (even if they are healthy foods), exercise more (as the overall physical condition allows), and be under the supervision of a qualified health-care provider. When we watch our diets and are mindful of calories and food quality, positive outcomes are right around the corner. We must also remember that we need an adequate amount of all the required nutrients and fluids for the body, and we need to remain active. With all other factors being equal, we are bound to lose the weight, stay fit, and enjoy a long and healthy life.

# CHAPTER 9

## The Dieting Approach in Addressing Obesity

By now, almost everyone is aware of the dangers posed by obesity. Not only does it affect our health, but it drains our resources and makes our children vulnerable to various threats to their well-being. Facing such an omen is not a choice; it is an obligation.

Currently, there is an obsession with dieting—that is an understatement. Depending on what statistic we are fond of, at any given moment in time, there is close to 40 percent of people on some kind of a diet. Everyone seems to be interested in losing weight, although recently, fewer Americans than ever claimed to be dieting. The overwhelming focus seems to be about finding the "miracle diet" that can take care of our weight issues once and for all. Unfortunately, this has yet to be discovered. Therefore, people use various methods to try to stay in shape. Some swear by a low-fat, low-protein, and high-carbohydrate diet; others believe in high fat, high protein and low carbohydrates, and the list goes on ad infinitum.

## The Medical Baseline

The first step toward dealing with overweight and obesity is to know our overall medical conditions. A certain percentage of people become overweight or obese because of some underlying medical conditions, such as hypothyroidism, glucose intolerance, depression, polycystic ovarian syndrome, Prader-Willi syndrome, and other inherited diseases. To determine which course of action to take, regardless of our genders and ages, we need to get a complete medical evaluation that includes a full physical examination, blood work, other testing based on our medical histories and complaints, and whatever subsequent work-up that may reveal any medical issues. This allows the qualified health-care provider to document any underlying conditions that may warrant medical treatment along with addressing our weight conditions.

BMI is an easy tool to assess whether a person is overweight or obese, although, as we have seen, it has its limitations. The formula is simple: (your weight in pounds is multiplied by 703, then that number is divided by your height in inches multiplied by itself (squared).

For example, a person is 175 pounds and five foot seven. First of all, convert the height to inches. Remember that 1 foot equals 12 inches, so 5 feet =equals 60 inches, then add another 7 inches, and the height is 67 inches. The formula will be to compute BMI is this: 175 × 703 = 123,025, then 123,025 / (67 × 67) = 27. The BMI would be twenty-seven.

With the result obtained, if the BMI is between twenty and twenty-five, then the person's weight is within normal limits; if it is between twenty-five and thirty, the person is overweight; if it is over thirty, the person is obese. From the example above, the BMI is twenty-seven, and therefore, that person would be overweight. When we look at the table, we must also consider age, gender, and height to determine ideal weight.

## The Diagnosis of Obesity

As we pointed out before, two-thirds of the population is overweight, and the person above is no exception. Based upon the percentage of weight, a patient is declared overweight (BMI 25–30) or obese (BMI above 30). The higher the BMI, the more overweight or obese a person is. Equally important is the distribution of body fat. The more fat that is laid down around your waist area (as opposed to hips), the higher your risk for obesity-related disease. Because weight loss is not easy, unless steps are taken in a timely manner, chances are the weight will keep rising. With age and other factors, the chance for influences on health and medical conditions also increases.

## An Efficient Way to Address Obesity

Once a diagnosis of overweight or obesity is made, the next step is to decide to overcome the condition by watching our two Qs: the quantity and the quality that go onto our plates.

### The Quantity

One of the fundamentals of dieting may be simple to state but more difficult to implement: restore the balance between our intake and consumed source of energy. In other words, to the best of our ability, see to it we use more energy than we consume by eating less.

### The Quality

When approaching the issue of weight management, the word *diet* does not seem to do justice to the concept. *Diet* in itself seems to evoke a pejorative connotation. It

JEAN D. FRANÇOIS MD

seems to suggest dying to normal life and becoming sad or withdrawn before our pitiful meal that we dare not enjoy. For many, it means restriction or resignation. It may signify fad dieting or ordering unregulated pills from overseas. To some, it may even mean starvation. This is not so at all!

The main idea is to take control of our lives in everything, including our nutritional consumption, to maintain good health throughout our lifetimes. We must recognize this as a long-term commitment to implement changes for healthy eating habits and daily physical activities while balancing calorie intake. In helping us reach the goal of a healthy weight, food plays an important part. Food is necessary to nourish us. It may even have the power to make us ill or cause premature death.

Our primary concern is to choose a practical variety of foods to meet our daily basic needs for nutrients to have enough energy to perform our daily activities. Our first step is to accept that our quantity and quality of foods need an evaluation to see what to keep and what to eliminate. To do so, we need to do the following:

1. *Find a reason* to change our weights, one that will motivate us to take the necessary steps to maximize the possibility for us to live healthier and longer lives.

2.  *Take inventory* of our daily eating habits and make a list that includes where and what we usually buy, where and how much we eat, and what is in our refrigerators.

3.  *Identify* the resources and healthier choices we need to make to get the best results.

4.  *Build* a list and have a bank of healthy foods on hand for a wide variety of choices.

5.  *Make a list* of physical activities and exercises that we enjoy. I may enjoy running. You may enjoy a game of basketball. We are all different.

6.  *Be willing* and motivated enough to face challenges, and be perseverant enough to stick to the plan. Also, be willing to make adjustments as we need to when we review our progress weekly.

7.  *Be true to ourselves* and do not let people dissuade us when it comes to doing what is right to stay healthy and keep the weight down; honestly look at the barriers to weight loss.

8.  *Realize* it is a lifetime commitment to keep our weights in check.

9.  *Remember* we are human beings; therefore, we may stumble or falter, but do not give up or be discouraged. We may even take a quick holiday for a special occasion, but be conscientious and refuse to turn back to the old way of eating.

10. *See* our weight conditions as a lifetime commitment that does not require a stringent, quick way of solving it but includes a combination of factors, including our overall attitudes, a genuine conception of life, and our ability to cope with the various earthly challenges. Therefore, be easy on ourselves. Identify ways to relax and enjoy this beautiful life.

11. *Learn* to appreciate ourselves and our efforts without being pompous or arrogant.

12. *Have one or more partners or a support group to join us*! Beware of the company you keep, as a supportive support system can make all the difference!

13. *Develop strategies* to keep the weight lost off for good.

We should get into the habit of discovering the secrets of those who have shed the weight and kept it off. These secrets include the following:

1. People who have lost weight are not obsessed with diets and dieting; they watch and control the portions of what they eat while remembering they are human and may indulge rarely without being dramatic about it.

2. Physical activities are an integral part of their lifestyles. They make fitness part of their daily routines.

3. They do not compete with others. They appreciate their successes as they come individually, yet they usually have support as well.

4. They keep good habits such as eating breakfast, drinking water, and respecting the tenet of six to eight hours of sleep each night.

## Types of Diets

We definitely need to explore the idea of diets further and figure out which one or which combination can work best. There are more than one hundred types of diets out there competing for our attention. *US News & World Report* has a list of the best diets,[12] where we can find some impressive information to help us in our choices. The following diets are cited: DASH, Mediterranean, MIND, Weight Watchers, Mayo Clinic, Volumetrics, Biggest Loser, Ornish, Abs, South Beach, Eco-Atkins, glycemic-index, Zone, raw food, Paleo, Jenny Craig, Atkins, SlimFast, beta HCG, gluten-free, and vegan diets. They were ranked according to the goal:

12  *US News & World Report*, 2017 Best Diets Rankings.

## Best Diets Overall
1. DASH diet
2. Mediterranean diet
3. MIND diet

## Best Commercial Diets
1. Mayo Clinic diet
2. Weight Watchers
3. Jenny Craig

## Best Weight-Loss Diets
1. Weight Watchers
2. Jenny Craig
3. Volumetrics

## Best Fast Weight-Loss Diets
1. HMR Program
2. Weight Watchers
3. Biggest Loser

## Best Diets for Healthy Eating
1. DASH diet
2. Mediterranean diet
3. MIND diet

**Easiest Diets to Follow**
1. Fertility diet
2. Mediterranean diet
3. MIND diet
4. Weight Watchers

**Best Diets for Diabetes**
1. DASH diet
2. Mediterranean diet
3. Vegan diet

**Best Diets for Heart Disease**
1. DASH diet
2. Ornish diet
3. TLC diet

**Best Plant-Based Diets**
1. Mediterranean diet
2. Flexitarian diet
3. Vegetarian diet

There are so many diets! If I did not mention them all, it is not because they are rejected or not good enough—it is simply because of the sheer number.

## Analysis of Available Diets

Which diet is healthier? Which one is detrimental to health?

The answer is not cut and dried. Depending on your goal, most of them tend to have a positive effect on those who are faithfully following them. Ideally, it would be great to identify a specific diet that has the magic formula to address all concerns, including weight loss, heart disease, stroke, brain cell protection, diabetes, aging, and cholesterol.

The ones closest to addressing these concerns seem to be the DASH and Mediterranean diets, for which there is evidence that following either will result in weight loss. However, the ideal diet has to be individualized with some fine tuning and adjustments here and there. There are pros and cons for all of them. Not one fits all, but the most successful reduces total energy intake.

Dieting is very popular, and it is important. This fast-and-furious approach usually has only short-term results, and some of these regimens can be detrimental to our health. The responsible approach is to adopt a balanced diet that is based on our overall medical conditions, genders, and ages. For a diet to be efficient, it needs to be part of our lifestyles and our daily standards of living. It must take into account how easily it can be followed and how cost effective and easily available it is. A gluten-free diet is not a low-fat diet. Many commercial gluten-free foods are high in fat and sugar (to replace the gluten), and if gluten-containing foods are replaced by a large quantity of rice and rice-containing foods, people may be in danger of ingesting excess arsenic, particularly if brown-rice syrup—even organic—is used as a sweetener. In addition, people following a gluten-free diet may have a higher risk for type 2 diabetes, possibly due to the low intake of fiber.

A diet should emphasize plant-based foods such as raw or lightly cooked vegetables, fruits, legumes, grains, nuts, seeds, along with some animal products such as organic lean meats, poultry, and fish and foods that are low in salt, fat, cholesterol, trans fats and saturated fats, and sugars. Everyone is different, but excessiveness or extremism does not help. The proper diet should avoid the monotony of a restricted list of tasteless foods. It is an individualized project that is reasonable and balanced and based on a variety of factors, including ancestral heritage, cultures, habits and beliefs, and psychosocial and environmental conditions.

## The Ketone-Based Diet

It is worth pointing out that there is an ongoing debate over ketones: are they the new energy source for the brain? A ketogenic diet includes high fat, moderate protein, and low (or no) carbs.

Ketones are made by the liver during fasting, starving, prolonged exercise, low carb diets, and untreated type 1 DM.

How important are ketones? They are water soluble—so they do not need lipoproteins or albumin to be carried through the body. They are produced in the liver when there are high levels of acetyl-CoA, which exceeds the oxidative capacity of the liver. During periods of fasting, the brain uses ketones to meet energy requirements. The low-carb/high-ketone diet is catching the attention of many scientific studies. The typical ketogenic diet, called the "long-chain triglyceride diet," provides three to four grams of fat for every one gram of carbohydrate and protein. In some studies it shows enhanced memory, clarity, attention, alertness, and cognition. The use of fatty acids breaks down into ketones as new fuel for the brain. Such a diet appears to be more efficient—fewer detrimental by-products are generated and less oxygen is needed, and therefore it works re efficiently. It has the ability to increase cellular respiration by increasing mitochondrial biogenesis, which increases metabolic efficiency.

In summary, a ketone-based diet for many is very promising. It has shown significant improvement theoretically and clinically and should be used as therapy for conditions such as intractable epilepsy, including glucose transporter type 1, pyruvate dehydrogenase deficiency,

Dravet syndrome, and Doose syndrome (myoclonic-astatic epilepsy).

Growing studies and benefits have been reported in severe and moderate Alzheimer's disease and hypoxic and ischemic brain injury—through mitochondrial function enhancement and rescuing of ATP for energy

Promising intervention in tumor growth and regeneration has also been proven in patients with not only CNS tumors but also gastric and genitourinary tumors.

Of course, more research and data are needed to grasp the extent of the benefits versus the risk for treatment or even prevention of certain diseases, including neurological conditions such as ALS, Parkinson's, autism, depression, and migraines. For further details, please refer to the ketogenic food pyramid.[13]


## Steps to Follow

The bottom line is that the type, content, and availability of the diet plays an important role in your compliance and ability to reach the targeted goal. Dietary

---

13 https://www.uptodate.com/contents/search?search=ketoneshttp://caloriesproper.com/ketosis-anti-brain-fog
https://www.ncbi.nlm.nih.gov/pubmed/23419562https://www.ruled.me/guide-keto-diet/
https://www.ruled.me/ketogenic-diet-food-list/ http://articles.mercola.com/sites/articles/archive/2016/09/04/ketogenic-nutritional-ketosis.aspx

recommendations may vary and may even seem conflicting for the common person looking for the right diet.

Like everything else in life, we need to invest time in our search and choice of food. It is important to take time to cook, or learn to cook, and to try different healthy foods with different recipes. It is beneficial to find ways and time to eat together with family members or friends. Our choice must be for the right kinds of foods that are high quality and well balanced with unprocessed, natural products.

Steps to reduce caloric intake:

- Search for foods with low calories (less energy-dense properties) like lean protein, fish, beans, fruits, vegetables, whole grains, and legumes.
- Adopt a balanced, multicolored diet with nutritious foods—the more color, the better!
- Obtain special plates and cups to measure portion sizes, or learn how much a portion size translates to common objects (e.g., one ounce equals one die; three ounces equals a deck of cards; one cup equals a baseball). Use smaller plates and bowls!
- In counting calories, remember to add those that come from dressings or other condiments. When eating out, be wary of the posted number

of calories listed per item; they are often not accurate and tend to be more than what is written.

- Avoid processed foods and even regular dairy products rich in fat and cholesterol. Instead, opt for low-fat products or milk alternatives.

- Pay attention to your drinks. Beware of the number of calories contained in each drink daily. Avoid sugary drinks. Sugar by any label or shape is still sugar (e.g., high-fructose corn syrup, maltodextrin, honey, brown sugar, molasses, dextrose, sucrose). Truvia and Splenda are noncaloric sweeteners, but studies conflict as to whether they are helpful for weight loss! Do not forget to drink a reasonable amount of sugar-free liquids daily. According to the Institute of Medicine, men should drink about thirteen cups (3 liters) of total fluids, and women should drink roughly nine cups (2.2 liters) of fluids daily (take care what you add into them). Remember that fruit juice may be "natural" but still contains sugar—check the label!

- Keep a log, or even take a picture, of what you eat daily; this is especially helpful with diabetics as one can look back and see which foods caused their glucose to spike. Take time to read nutrition labels and the ingredients in what you are consuming. The ingredient that is listed first is the ingredient that weighs the most in the product. If you are looking to buy whole-wheat bread, make sure the first ingredient listed is whole wheat and not refined/processed flour (the front of the packaging will usually state 100 percent whole-wheat bread). Do not be fooled by packaging or the color of the product.

- Be very particular about your snacks. They should be made up of fruits, low-fat yogurt, nuts, and raw vegetables while keeping an eye on the sugar content.

- Have a weekly meal plan with the detailed three main meals daily and an average three snacks or even a light supper. When you go grocery shopping, stick to buying only the items on your list. It is also helpful not to go grocery shopping when you are hungry as this may lead you to wanting to buy everything in your path!

- Do not be afraid to bring along your own meals to work if you feel the environment is not conducive to making healthy choices.

- Avoid eating late at night and going to bed immediately following dinner. It will not only mess with restful sleep but will affect your digestive health. Also, take your time to chew your food. People who eat slower and chew more tend to be more in touch with their hunger/satiety cues. Try putting down your utensil in between bites.

- Plan to follow a plant-based diet using animal protein as a flavoring tool, not the main part of the meal.

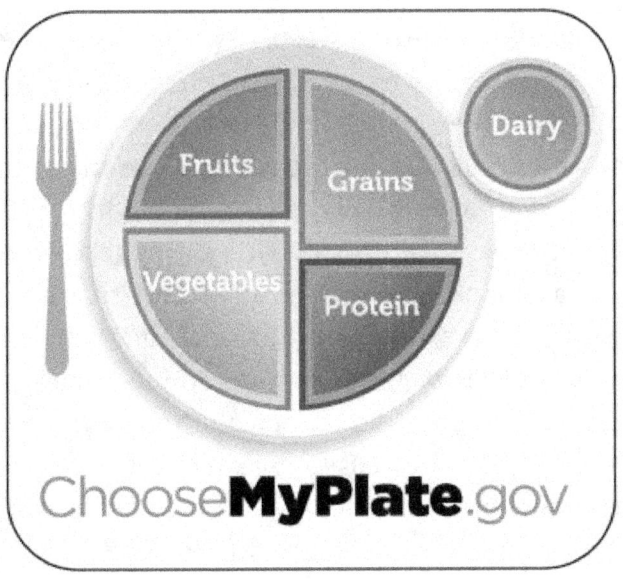

## To Be or Not to Be... Vegan?

In an interview with Joe Conason and published in the magazine *AARP*, President Clinton stated, "I decided to pick the diet that I thought would maximize my chances of long-term survival." It is reported that through such a diet, the forty-second president of the United States lost thirty pounds and has managed to stay in shape since then. This is a very eloquent testimony in favor of a vegan diet. As many of us embark on improved ways and means to maximize our energy and our healing capacities as well as stay fit and healthy, it is worth considering the vegan diet.

There is a difference between vegetarian and vegan diets. Without splitting hairs, vegetarians are people who do not consume meat, fish, or poultry. They eat fruits, vegetables, grains, and seeds. Some vegetarians consume eggs and dairy products; some may not eat them. They do not usually eat products with gelatin or other meat-based products. However, those who adhere to a vegan diet adopt a philosophy that excludes all foods of animal origin or the use of animals for clothing or any other purpose. In a vegan diet, many fruits, vegetables, legumes, seeds, cereals, and nuts are consumed. They may even use soybean products to replace their dairy products.

It is worth noting that those who are very strict in such a diet may run the risk of being deficient in iron, iodine, vitamin B12, calcium, vitamin D, and omega-3s. I know someone who at around thirteen years of age decided she would become a vegetarian. We will never know if that inhibited or aided in her growth as a young person. She persisted in that lifestyle up until adulthood. Then she decided to make the leap to a vegan lifestyle. She fell ill during that year. She was deficient in vitamin A, omega-3s, and even vitamin D! Her enthusiasm was derailed when she decided to eat meat for her health. Not everyone has a similar experience though. We need to be careful as to how we obtain all the necessary nutrients to stay healthy when following such a restrictive diet.

Some of the strictest followers are vegan for their faiths and religious convictions. To those people, I would say make sure you consult with a qualified physician who know or even share your faith, who can refer you to a registered dietitian, who will advise you how to choose foods to avoid deficiencies, and if a deficiency occurs, how to address it immediately.

Otherwise, most people prefer a vegetarian diet because it helps to lose the pounds and to keep them off while obtaining essential nutrients through egg or seafood consumption. If in the beginning, you do not feel comfortable enough to make that drastic 180-degree turn to adopt a vegan or vegetarian diet, you can start slow by cutting back on the portion size and type and frequency of meat consumption and gradually cut meat out of your diet. The plant-based diet has been shown to be health conducive while not being too restrictive. If you adopt this diet, see your doctor regularly, have a plan, and use supplements when recommended. It is usually good to avoid all extremes, and dieting is no exception.

## On Skipping Breakfast

Because we are always pressed for time, we try our best to find some efficient shortcut to reach our goals. Nevertheless, skipping breakfast to cut calories does not necessarily cut it. When we wake up, our stomachs are empty and in dire need of some food.

1.  If we rush out to work or to take care of our daily activities without eating, we are functioning on a low level of energy to face life's daily challenges. Remember, bodies need a certain percentage of energy for breathing, blinking, and pumping blood. If we begin our days with a bare minimum of nutrients, our bodies receive a signal to activate the backup plan for a possible famine. Our metabolisms slow down. Even if we are active, we will burn fewer calories in such a condition, and our bodies will store more fat. In addition, the body's metabolism is fastest in the morning.

2.  During the day, eventually we will experience hunger. This can lead to spontaneous grabbing of unhealthy snacks or a large meal at lunchtime that is likely to be much bigger than the ideal portion, forcing increased storage.

3.  When we fast for many hours and then eat a considerable portion of food, the pancreas

tends to respond by producing the corresponding amount of insulin to meet the increased amount of glucose in our systems. The insulin should allow the sugar (glucose) in the blood to transfer to the body's cells to be stored as glycogen, which will then be used by the cells for energy (after being converted to adenosine triphosphate), and then the body will reestablish the equilibrium.

In contrast, according to a study recently presented by Dr. Elizabeth Thomas (instructor of medicine at the University of Colorado School of Medicine), for a small number of women, after skipping who skip breakfast, the body's cells required more insulin to absorb the glucose, whose level remained significantly high. Although the research was small and the observation was temporary, it is worth considering while further studies are being pursued.

The prudent step is to have a nutritious, balanced breakfast with fiber and protein to keep us full and strong for the rest of the day. Again, researchers reveal that eating breakfast helps us to have a more stable weight. Start the day off on the right foot; eat a healthy breakfast! Beware of breakfast cereals though, as many are high in sugar and made of processed grains. If you like breakfast cereals, choose those whose first ingredient is whole grain.[14]

Bottom line: if you are not a breakfast eater, try to eat a substantial snack as soon as you can in the first part of the day.

Bear in mind that not all the data are collected to give us a full grasp about obesity. Actually, a new study by a team under the leadership of David Allison, PhD, of the University of Alabama failed to prove the direct link between skipping breakfast and obesity. The bottom line is that more research needs to be done. But it is safe to say that when we are hungry or feel like we are starving, we are less choosy in the quality and quantity of foods we eat.

## Is There Wiggle Room?

One of the concerns many people have is that dieting will feel as if their lives are ending. This is far from the truth! You can still go out and dine with friends. You can still eat dessert! You can still visit fast-food restaurants, although not as often as before. Take a look at the menu, and find

---

14  Thomas, E. A., J. Higgins, D. H. Bessesen, B. McNair, and M. A. Cornier, "Usual breakfast eating habits affect response to breakfast skipping in overweight women." *Obesity.* (2015) doi: 10.1002/oby.21049.

some healthy choices. Nowadays, even fast-food places have salads or grilled chicken or some form of lean meat. The key is to remain committed to being health conscious and making exercise a part of your daily routines.

## Should You Join a Weight-Loss Program?

Once we make the decision to keep our weights in check, we should be willing to take all the necessary steps to be successful at it. After all, the fringe benefits include a general sense of well-being, an improvement in some medical conditions, and ultimately, longevity and a sense of personal satisfaction. So, the first approach is to acquire enough knowledge to be able to do it on your own. You can also get one or two people to join you. The road to weight loss is easier when we do it with others. However, alone or with others, if the acquired knowledge is not giving us the results we expected or if we have reached a plateau, then we should consider joining a weight-loss program.

## Criteria to Consider in Choosing a Weight-Loss Program

There are many instances in which to overcome the challenges of obesity or being overweight, people need to take some more aggressive steps to lose the weight. One way to do that is to join a weight-loss program. There are so many of them. You should choose a weight-loss program that meets the following criteria:

- Is medically supervised
- Aids you in setting realistic goals for yourself
- Has an integrative approach to your weight condition and does basic work-up: history and physical, blood work, electrocardiogram, and any other tests that are necessary
- Proposes meal planning and calorie control
- Takes time and encourages patience
- Proposes proper exercise and includes coaching
- Has variety in the diet
- Has a maintenance program
- Is not greedy or money hungry but instead is interested in your health and well-being

Along with considering our genetic packages, diets, levels of exercise, and BMRs, we also need to consider some instances for detoxification to eliminate waste and toxins from our system. The ways of detoxifying or removing toxins can be simple through the foods consumed. Yes, more fruits, vegetables, legumes, and whole grains promote laxation. Some examples of cleansing foods include wild rice, brussels sprouts, cabbage, carrot, papaya, peaches, cauliflower, and celery, along with water intake. Foods that are high in insoluble fiber tend to increase the bulk of our stool, thus "cleaning out" our colons. Just make sure to have adequate fluid intake when increasing the amount of fiber in your diet. Also, slowly increase the amount of fiber to avoid unpleasant symptoms such as increased gas and bloating.

Foods such as green, leafy vegetables like kale and cabbage, and some fruits such as apples, tomatoes, lemons, grapes, plums, and oranges play a positive role in keeping us healthy. The same goes for regular exercises, drinking water, and the proper state of mind. They play a significant role in keeping us healthy. Again, a whole package acts harmoniously to maintain a healthy condition.

# CHAPTER 10

Physical Activities to Tackle Obesity

Overcoming obesity requires a number of things. Besides counting calories, we must also take inventory of our levels of physical activity. In general, the idea of physical activity is cardinal proof that we are still alive. Any movements performed that involve the use of our muscles can be counted as part of physical activity. Routine daily household tasks, walking from one room to another, and housecleaning are all examples of general physical activity.

Exercise for weight loss is a more intentional decision that involves repetitive action to stay in shape and be physically fit. It can include activities such as brisk walking, resistance-band exercises, heavy gardening, lawn mowing, jogging, swimming, climbing, hiking, biking, skiing, and weight training using barbells, dumbbells, or weight machines. Depending on our overall medical conditions, to stay fit, we should aim for moderate to vig-orous, systematic, planned activities that will benefit our hearts and provide muscular strength and flexibility for our overall well-being. The length of time and the inten-sity needs to be taken into account. The recommended amount is about half to one hour of moderate to vigor-ous programmed exercise daily. Although exercise has be-come more and more popular lately, we must admit it is not easy to keep up. We are always pressed for time, and our obligations pull us in different directions. As a matter of fact, the reported data suggest that far less than 30 per-cent of the population makes exercise part of their daily plans.

Many people are afraid to begin a formal exercise pro-gram because they do not realize that they do not have to compete with the professional athletes. Instead, we need to find ways to implement exercise into our schedules, however creative it has to be. I have often seen new par-ents running with baby strollers in the park or including the babies into their workouts.

Furthermore, if we really want to lose weight and stay fit, we cannot starve ourselves. There is a limit on how many calories we can cut from our daily diets. The rest of our weight-loss journeys must include exercise. The best way is to start slow and increase progressively according to our overall physical conditions.

Generally, an average of thirty minutes of moderate aerobic activity should be part of the regular daily routine; a total of one hundred fifty minutes weekly should do the trick. Those who can go for vigorous aerobic activity or a mix of moderate and vigorous aerobic activity routines can make the proper adjustment in time spent per activity. If you can play sports or join a gym, do it! Some of us may only be able to do a regular walk or perform regular household chores; if these are the only things you can do, go ahead and do them. The key is to stay active and improve your health. Start by walking and taking the stairs when it is feasible. Try interacting with children or grandchildren. Children are always moving! No matter what, keep your body moving—it is essential to life!

Exercise is good for us all. It is good for children, good for men and women, and good for the elderly. It helps us burn calories to stay in shape. The key is to vary the activities based on your age group, your needs, and your medical condition. The result is an individual endeavor that depends on the weight and overall physical condition and shape of the participant and the frequency, amount of time spent, type, and speed at which the exercise is done. It helps us to keep our weights in check.

Exercise also helps combat and improve conditions such as cancer, hypertension, heart disease, high cholesterol, stroke, diabetes, and osteoporosis. Exercise keeps us flexible and strengthens our joints and muscles. It also gives us an overall sense of well-being, helps us cope with stress, and improves our cognitive function. Exercising will help our physiological ages be less than our chronological ages—who does not want to age gracefully?

## Twelve Easy Steps for a Rewarding Exercise Period

1. *Be willing and motivated to do it!* Do not say you will exercise for one hour and quit after thirty minutes.
2. *Have a specific plan.* Set realistic short-term and long-term goals.
3. *Get some basic tools.* Gather a comfortable pair of sneakers, loose clothes comfortable enough to protect you against the cold in wintertime and keep you cool in the summer, a water bottle, a musical device, and a pedometer or a fitness tracker such as the Fitbit. There are so many options available!
4. *Choose activities you enjoy.* If you abhor running, do not start training for a marathon. The idea is to do something you enjoy so you feel motivated to stick with it.

5.  *Start walking at a leisurely pace.* Do it for fifteen or thirty minutes in your neighborhood, at work, or wherever you feel safe.

6.  *Try using public transportation.* If there is reasonably safe and regular public transportation from home to work or school, park the car and give it a try! Going up the steps or walking on the subway platform will count. Try it for one week and see the results. You may feel strange or tired at the beginning, but the more you do it, the more stamina you will build. The best part is you will be able to get in shape without having to put aside special time to work out and sweat. At the end of the day, you will be surprised to see the results. If you are like me, this will become an incentive for you to walk at every chance you have in your neighborhood, climb the stairs instead of waiting for the elevator, and stand and take a few steps every now and then. Every little bit counts and adds up.

7.  *Try to vary the menu.* Bicycling, dancing, gardening, jogging, going to the gym, walking in a park, running on the neighborhood track, swimming, playing tennis, playing racquetball, jumping rope, hiking, lifting weights, or playing basketball are

all activities you can try. Practicing one or two of these activities daily for about thirty minutes or more should help you burn between 150 and 250 calories. So if you lose 1,500 calories per week in exercise and another 2,000 in dieting, making a total of 3,500 calories, all other factors being equal, you should lose about one pound per week. Over time, adjustments will be needed, but you will be in the swing of losing and maintaining a healthy weight instead of gaining or dangerously starving yourself through a crash diet.

8. *Pick your own pace.* If physical activity and exercise are to be part of a long-term commitment, you cannot be competing with anyone. Just be consistent and persevere.

9. *Be sociable.* Have a support group made up of family members and friends. Pick people with whom you get along well—not those who will become an additional source of stress.

10. *Beware of excuses.* Do not say, "I'm too tired," "I do not have enough time," "I have too much to do," and "I am too shy to go to the gym where everyone is looking at me." You do not have to go to the gym. Allow yourself no excuses. Start slow but venture out and do it.

11. *Adjust your types of activities by day and season.* Some will be indoors; others will be outdoors. The key is to have a program of exercise.
12. *Remember, you can start at any age.* All of us stand to benefit from exercise, and it is never too late to start. Procrastination and good intention alone do not count.

## Precautions

Remember, the goal is to stay fit and healthy. It is paramount that exercise is done safely—warming up, stretching, starting slowly, and moving up according to what you can tolerate. Overdoing it may cause torn muscles or ligaments, soreness, fatigue, or other injuries or diseases. You should always seek the advice of your physician.

If you are older than forty-five, smoke, are obese, or have chronic medical conditions or a family history of heart conditions, you must get clearance from your doctor, who will tell you the type and the limit of exercise you can perform. All of us can be physically active. The key is to consider what kind, how much, and for how long. If there is any doubt, always check with your doctor, who may refer you to a cardiologist for further work-up before clearing you for an exercise routine.

# CHAPTER 11

## Combating Obesity:
## Bullets to Load Your Gun

B
y now, we know that obesity is multifactorial; therefore, it is important to have a multidisciplinary approach to address the different causes and fight such a disease. In our journeys to better health and weight control, adopting healthy food consumption and regular exercise can become a habit. By adopting such a pattern of behavior as a permanent new lifestyle, we can have a better handle on our weights and improve our health and our overall well-being. Such an approach may be easier for some than others. Often, people find in foods some comfort not found elsewhere. Overeating becomes a coping mechanism to deal with stress; rejection; boredom; familial, emotional, and chemical imbalances; and societal issues.

Food is a source of comfort for many who tell themselves they deserve to eat as much as they want. All kinds of unhealthy choices are appealing to them to reward themselves for all their hard work or even rare accomplishments. Sometimes this concept is passed down from generation to generation. Your parents may have rewarded themselves with an ice cream or a couple of cocktails every day after work, so you do the same. Another family member may have indulged in cake after finishing an important project, so every time you sell a house, you head to Dairy Queen. Furthermore, parties never lack food and drinks and usually include alcohol and smoking. This is why behavioral modification and exploring coping mechanisms are part of the overall approach of how to effectively deal with obesity.

## 1. Behavioral modification

Behavior modification is a tool used to aid in the fight against obesity. To succeed, you must do the following:

- Recognize the specific problem, and identify the causes (diet, types of foods, availability, frequency, and amount).
- It is not mandatory to focus on counting calories because it may be overwhelming for many people; instead, you can focus on making small changes in the types of foods you choose, one at a time.

For example, first eliminate sugar-sweetened beverages, then work on eating a balanced breakfast, then focus on adding more fiber and vegetables into your diet.

- Identify stressors and work to eliminate, cope with, or ameliorate them!

- Consider your lifestyle (use of drugs, alcohol, and tobacco), your mental state, thought process, and your self-image.

- Establish goals (the advantages and disadvantages of a change on the current state of health), gauge your level of motivation, and make a decision to change.

- Establish a protocol/plan. Know when, where, and how to implement the decisions and new measures for food and activities, and act on them.

- Seek support when needed; find a support network.

- No matter what, you can do it. You deserve it!

In these sessions, you can also find out if you really want to lose weight. Sometimes a patient loves his disease—that is to say, the patient is familiar with the current condition that provides certain benefits such as care and attention received from other members of the household or members of the community only because of the situation. People may be afraid of losing such attention once they are doing better. They may not be ready to shoulder their responsibilities. All this must be taken into consideration and may interfere with weight-loss measures that involve a change in lifestyle.

## 2. Environment

In terms of obesity, environment is defined as one of the various factors that determines our lifestyles and results in a negative or positive effect on our weight. Besides our eating habits, housing placement can also influence our health status and impede or facilitate our health. An unhealthy house may have lead, dust, mold, and roaches that can cause allergies or trigger asthma and eczema. An unsafe neighborhood may keep everyone in the house, which leads to a sedentary lifestyle. No one dares to venture out; therefore, there is lack of physical activity, which has a negative effect on weight and fitness. A neighborhood or community devoid of any parks, gyms, proper lighting, sidewalks, and safe transportation may have a negative effect on behavior, health, and fitness. The proper environment should provide supermarkets where healthy foods are available at an affordable price. The workplace, type of school, supermarket, and urban design all contribute to encouraging or discouraging healthy behavior and an active lifestyle.

This leads us to the conclusion that the fight against obesity should deeply involve the leaders of this country and the world. To overcome obesity and sustain a healthy lifestyle for all, there must be a conjoined effort from the private sectors, corporations, schools, media, communities, religious leaders, and elected officials to foster policies that address issues such as health equity and food access as well as social justice and prevention or intervention against gangs and other reckless behaviors that are prejudicial to health. We must stop practicing reactive health care, adopt a proactive approach, and create effective strategies that encourage prevention.

## 3. Genetics and hormonal changes

Scientific research supports the fact that genetic predisposition plays a role in obesity. As a matter of fact, certain medical disorders are directly related to genes. In reality, we need to remember that our genetic compositions do not change. And our physical makeups will not change overnight. Because obesity has been plaguing us at an alarming rate only in the last few decades, we cannot blame it completely on genes. Nevertheless, it is a contributor, and we must address it.

Usually, because of several factors, as we age, we tend to gain weight. The changes are often more drastic and more difficult to control in women than men. Most of the weight challenges for women come around the peri-menopausal/menopausal time. Hormonal fluctuations and an imbalance in estrogen, progesterone, testosterone, and cortisol play a role. The reasonable approach is to investigate the hormonal levels and address the changes by adopting hormonal replacement to reestablish the balance. A natural approach is advised as much as possible. Nevertheless, we need to be aware of the reported side effects of hormonal replacement. After deciding whether we want to go for hormonal replacement, diligent research is required to determine how to replace them.

## 4. Sleeping

In our quest to get our weights under control, we must turn every single stone. Let us look at our sleeping habits. In a world in which we are generally very busy and have so many gadgets at our disposal, it is common for many to sacrifice sleep to perform other tasks such as work that was not completed during the day. You may also be a night worker with limited ability to sleep during the day. You may stay up late to watch TV or text or talk on the phone. I read something some time ago: "Good night,

Dad, but I really mean I'm going to lay prone and play on my phone." This is not healthy.

There have been several studies supporting the relationship between sleep and health risks in general and weight gain in particular. Staying up when we should be asleep affects our metabolism function and causes hormonal changes, including an increased level of the hormone that stimulates our appetites, ghrelin, and a decrease in the hormone that is supposed to suppress our appetites and make us feel full, leptin. This leads to an increased sensation of hunger, food consumption, and poor self-control in our choice of foods. Sleep-deprived people tend to feel tired and sluggish; they show impaired judgment, have difficulty exercising, and are more susceptible to some diseases such as diabetes. Furthermore, a lack of sleep can affect growth hormones, decrease metabolic rate and even growth in children, cause gluttony, increase snacking and consumption of inappropriate foods, and affect the appetite- controlling hormones. Sleep hygiene is important. It aids with weight management. Therefore, one of the effective steps to overcome obesity is to address the quantity and the quality of our sleep. [15]

---

15 Breuss, Michael, PhD, and Debra Fulghum Bruce, PhD; *The Sleep Doctor's Diet Plan*

Key factors for a meaningful sleep pattern include the following:

1. Have regular hours for sleep.
2. Sleep for six to eight hours daily.
3. Eliminate or reduce noise and light where you sleep (be aware that the light from device screens affects the body's ability to fall sleep).
4. Avoid certain activities before sleep—for example, scary movies, disturbing news, loud music, or exciting books are not bedtime activities.
5. Turn off the phone ringer, if feasible.
6. Stay away from checking your e-mail, Twitter feed, or any other social media.
7. Beware of the restless, noisy partner sharing your bed.
8. Stay off the bed and be active during the day. This means you can read at a desk or in the living room or kitchen but not in bed!
9. Avoid daily naps if they affect your ability to sleep at night.
10. See your doctor for any underlying sleep problem, including sleep apnea. Avoid sleep medications as much as possible.

Studies remain ongoing as scientists aim to find and explain the correlation between sleep and weight gain. Until then, suffice it to say that sleep deprivation negatively affects our ability to keep our weights under control.

## 5. Stress management and obesity

This is a competitive world. We face stress everywhere and at any time. Although we need a certain level of stress to function at our best to make important decisions, we must return to our homeostatic state. More often than not, we face constant stressful situations, psychosocial fears, and anxiety that have a negative effect on our well-being by affecting our nervous systems, our immune systems, and our endocrine systems. As a matter of fact, researchers have found that increased and persistent stress leads us to make poor food choices because we are looking for comfort foods that are usually high in sugar, fats, and calories. Stress increases the serotonin level to comfort you in your stressful situation. Active stressors put us in fight-or-flight mode (more fight that flight), which triggers an increased release of cortisol that fosters increased fat absorption and has a negative effect on our food choices and eating habits. Researchers are working to find a way to reverse or block stress-induced obesity by blocking neuropeptide Y, a neuropeptide molecule from the nerve cells that has a special affinity for certain fat cell receptors to facilitate fat cell accumulation and development. Usually those stressors in our lives are nonphysical; they are emotional, psychological, or even sociocultural in a global economy.

We may still be working to find ways to fight obesity, but scientific studies lead us to believe that stress is one of the components. Because stress has become an integral part of our daily lives, and because it is not likely to go away, it is imperative we find ways to manage our stress instead of being managed by stress.

The following are thirteen simple steps to deal with stress:

1. Identify the stressors and their sources; do not deny their existence.
2. Gauge the effects of stress based on your perception and overall well-being (e.g., personality, character, internal/personal issues, developed coping mechanism, self-esteem, psychosocial issues)
3. Learn to identify priorities, such as deadline versus routine.

4. Develop skills to identify the upcoming stressful situations, the stressful environment, and the toxic personalities around you. Plan accordingly.
5. Do not procrastinate.
6. Be disciplined.
7. Be willing to learn from past mistakes instead of being paralyzed by them.
8. Have a positive attitude coupled with diligence.
9. Have a plan of action and be realistic.
10. Find ways to relax.
11. Build a supportive network of family and friends.
12. Surround yourself with healthy foods and snacks.
13. Remember, if all else fails, there is no permanent condition. Every situation is temporary; we are only human. This too shall pass!

## 6. Water has been shown to help curb obesity

Because people who are overweight and obese retain water, some people tend to associate water intake with weight gain. But unless there is some underlying medical condition that warrants fluid restriction, drinking a significant amount of potable water daily is an excellent way to help with weight loss. Very often, what is perceived as hunger is, in fact, thirst. Water is a very important component of our bodies. As a matter of fact, it makes up 60–70 percent of our body weights. Drinking the right amount of water must be part of our daily routines. It goes through our bodies to bring along nutrients to our cells, and it flushes toxins out of our organs. This immediately brings up two major questions: How much water should we drink? Can we ever drink too much water?

The quantity of water that we should drink usually depends on each individual. Based on gender, the safe range is between nine and thirteen eight-ounce glasses of fluid (2.2 liters for women; 3 liters for men), primarily and preferably potable water to make the urine a pale straw color. It is recommended to drink water before each meal and between regular meals, upon awakening in the morning, and before going to bed. Obviously, factors such as weather, types and frequency of exercise, lifestyle, medical conditions, breastfeeding, and pregnancy have an effect if adjusting the quantity of liquids to drink.

When we drink water first, we satisfy our thirst, and that decreases our hunger, making the stomach feel a bit less empty and therefore much more prone to feel full with less food. Water helps to flush out the toxins in our systems and brings needed nutrients to our cells.

A few words of caution—avoid taking in too much water; drinking an amount that is more than needed at a fast rate and within a short time span may affect the level of sodium (an electrolyte) in the body. This is why it is recommended to stay within the mentioned norms and consult with a doctor to avoid either dehydration or water intoxication.

Further studies are being done to shed more light on the positive effects of water consumption and weight loss.

## 7. Love, sex, relationships, and obesity

Responsible, legitimate relationships in which love and intimacy blossom, can play a positive role in pursuing and maintaining the ideal weight. As a matter of fact, intimate, responsible, and consensual relationships make the partners feel good, and they nurture one another. Sex burns calories, which helps your daily calorie budget. It also helps psychologically, making you forget the burdens of daily life and helping you sleep better and relax.

## 8. Holistic approach to weight loss

The holistic approach is an integrated approach in which all aspects of life are taken into consideration to allow the person to make necessary choices. This is the starting point for appropriate changes to reach the desired lifestyle with support and guidance. The holistic approach is also called *holistic medicine*. It encompasses the body, mind, and soul. All of these parts of us are essential in maintaining our health.

Let us consider for a moment the following example: You go to a restaurant with your child. While your family is eating fruits and vegetables, the customer at the next table is eating a large, juicy, and delicious hamburger with french-fries and a large Coke. Most likely, you will notice a change in your child's facial expression. The person who is eating that high-fat, salty meal with a sugary drink seems to be happy. Once your son glances at him, he may wish he had that hamburger and look a little sad. When the only argument you have is to tell him we eat healthy and green foods to maintain good health, do you think he will listen to you? By nature, we want whatever looks good now. We want to feel great when we eat, even if appearances are deceiving. However, the earlier we start, the better off we are. In fact, when we are first introducing foods to babies, we want to start with unseasoned vegetables and fruits so that they come to love and accept the natural tastes of these foods. If children have never eaten a high-fat, high-salt meal with a soda, they will not miss it.

## 9. The macro approach to controlling obesity

Because obesity has multiple causes, it also requires a number of measures to tackle the condition. As indicated above, there are other factors to consider to obtain relevant data on the obesity crisis. Food sources must be regulated and monitored. The government should provide clear guidelines and put in place a structure for the enforcement of healthy recommendations. It must also be the duty of the state to make healthy food more easily accessible, adjust the prices of food, educate the population, and project a new attitude that champions healthy lifestyles in general and healthy eating habits in particular. The Healthy, Hunger-Free Kids Act signed by President Obama and championed by Michelle Obama is a step in the right direction—teaching healthy eating habits to children will ensure they are off to a healthy start in life. However, more needs to be done at the local, state, and national levels!

There is a conflict of interest between a booming sector that produces unhealthy foods and the government that needs to regulate these industries. Public health is threatened due to the consumption of these foods that ultimately make people sick as well as driving up the cost of health care. There is a need for greater regulation of food advertising (especially to children) and companies who make unsubstantiated health claims on their products. How much of the obesity crisis should the individual be responsible for? We may not want the government to play Big Brother, and yet it does not look as though an individual's will power will fix the situation. (Consider the extent of individual freedom, the role of prescription drugs, and surgery micro/macro structural interaction a lack of sleep can affect growth hormones, decrease metabolic rate and even growth in children, cause gluttony, increase snacking and consumption of inappropriate foods, and affect the appetite- controlling hormones. Sleep hygiene is important. It aids with weight management. Therefore, one of the effective steps to overcome obesity is to address the quantity and the quality of our sleep..) The food supply is currently subsidized, weighted *against* healthful fruits and vegetables and small farmers and *for* the products of agribusiness (e.g., soybeans and corn) and large farmers. There needs to be a revision in government policy regarding the national agricultural approach, and it needs to be geared toward the health of the nation and not toward special interests aimed at making profits. It is time for fruits and vegetables to be less expensive and more easily accessible everywhere. Furthermore, the way we raise livestock in the United States needs to be looked at and regulated—do we really want to be eating beef and poultry that are injected with hormones and raised in unsanitary conditions? Yes, we have options, but those better options are usually much more expensive.

Cost and availability are big factors that influence people's choices. This explains why there is a trend toward adding taxes to unhealthy foods and beverages, affecting the volume of drinks and the amount of junk foods purchased. Certain countries in Europe have already adopted this tax on unhealthy foods such as sugar-sweetened beverages and saturated fats. This thought process is similar to the one that caused the price of tobacco to go up—make it so expensive that consumers will not purchase it. Those advocating for such an approach are hoping that an increased cost for unhealthy foods and beverages may sway people and cause them to switch to healthier choices that will cost less. But people may choose to pay extra for their junk foods, or the manufacturers and retailers may choose to absorb the tax penalty. There is evidence already from California and Mexico that it is working. No matter what, the health of the population should always be the goal when creating and implementing policies.

## Overall Attitude

Obesity involves all of us. It affects individuals, family members, extended family members, and communities and requires implementing appropriate policies and making changes tactfully. Eating should be a healthy as well as a pleasurable experience.

Many people are concerned about obesity, but few people have found the ideal solution—even among those who seem to have gotten a handle on it. Weight loss does not seem to last for long, so many people's weight goes like a yo-yo. The rate of people returning to previous eating habits, or even worse than before, remains high, although according to the National Weight Registry, some people do succeed. Have discipline and flexibility. Persevere, plan, and interact with others on the same path as much as possible. Watch out for procrastination or complaining. They do not help.

# CHAPTER 12

## Role of Medication and Surgery in Treating Obesity

### Medication

Not everyone is going to change from a size sixteen to a size eight through diet and exercise alone. Everyone is different; it depends on your age, size, weight, behavior, medical conditions, genetics, environment, and level of activity. There are instances when besides healthy eating and exercise, a competent physician may recommend certain medications. Antiobesity drugs are available that suppress appetite, increase metabolism, or block fat absorption and help us lose weight. However, we must be careful and read the labels for side effects. We should take medicine only if conservative treatment does not work and while under the supervision of a qualified physician who has to obtain a thorough medical, allergies, and family history background and also perform a thorough exam before starting the medication. While on the medication, you must have routine checkups and testing on a regular basis.

We cannot be cavalier about popping pills here and there while continuing to follow an irresponsible lifestyle that is nonconducive to weight loss. If we smoke, eat food indiscriminately, and do not exercise, then the medications may not be as effective as they should be; plus, there are side effects that go with all medications. Before starting a weight-loss medication, your physician must determine if the benefits outweigh the risks. It must be a comprehensive plan that combines a healthy, balanced diet with the percentage of carbohydrates, proteins, and fats that work for you.

The US Department of Health and Human Services has provided guidelines as to when medications should be used to lose weight:

- The BMI is thirty or more, or the BMI is twenty-seven or more with conditions such as hypertension, high cholesterol, or type 2 diabetes.
- The use of medications is for a short-term basis. The weight loss is generally noted in the first three to six months. The continuation of the medication beyond that may not be as effective

as initially and may even cause weight gain in some instances.

- The outcome depends on the patient's overall condition, the medication, and the patient's adherence.
- Beware of side effects that can be quite significant—for example, headaches, dizziness/giddiness, stomach discomfort, diarrhea, constipation, nausea, dry mouth, changes in sleep habits, nervousness, stuffy nose, restlessness, tingling, numbness of hands and feet, increased heart rate, increased blood pressure, changes in taste, and blurred vision. Overall, the side effects vary with each medication, the dosage, and the individual level of adjustment and tolerance. They tend to be mild and diminish if the patient continues to take the medication under a doctor's supervision. Medications are usually not advised for children and elderly. They are sometimes labeled "controlled substances" because of the potential for addiction and abuse.

The government agency that reviews medications to be prescribed in the United States is the Food and Drug Administration (FDA). The FDA has approved a few medications to be used in case of obesity. They include the following:

1. Orlistat (Xenical) has been around since 1999. It works by blocking the enzyme lipase (lipase inhibitor), which usually breaks down the fat. So, on average, one-third of the fat from ingested food is stopped from being absorbed. When less fat is broken down to be processed, fewer calories are taken in, causing the weight loss. Patients who take Orlistat may lose between 5 and 10 percent of their weight while consuming a diet that is low in calories and fat. Orlistat's prescribed dosage is one hundred twenty milligrams (Xenical), or the over-the-counter version is sixty milligrams and is called Alli, which is not approved for use by children. Orlistat can be taken up to three times a day or less with fat-containing meals. Users of Orlistat should also be prescribed multivitamin supplements due to the risk of decreased absorption of fat-soluble vitamins.

2. Phentermine-Topiramate (Qsymia) is a combination of two separate medications: phentermine, known to suppress appetite, and a lack of sleep can affect growth hormones, decrease metabolic rate and even growth in children, cause gluttony,

increase snacking and consumption of inappropriate foods, and affect the appetite- controlling hormones. Sleep hygiene is important. It aids with weight management. Therefore, one of the effective steps to overcome obesity is to address the quantity and the quality of our sleep. Topiramate, which is used for seizures and migraines. The two together is called Qsymia, which was approved by the FDA in July 2012 (though not universally approved around the world) to be used as long-term weight-loss medicine. It is on formulary in three doses and is available with a prescription through certified pharmacies. Patients with recent heart conditions or stroke; who are pregnant; who have hyperthyroidism, glaucoma, or suicidal tendency; or who use certain types of antidepressants should not take Qsymia.

3. Lorcaserin hydrochloride (Belviq) was also approved by the FDA in June 2012. It works by causing a sensation of fullness via the chemicals in the brain (serotonin activation). Once the patient feels full, he or she is less likely to continue eating.

Other drugs have been approved by the FDA for only a short duration, not to go beyond twelve weeks. They include phentermine, phendimetrazine, diethylpropion, and benzphetamine. They are available under various names.

The bottom line is that prescribed weight-loss medication can work in combination with proper diet and exercise. Because the research behind these medications is limited and recent, prudence is in order while taking any of them. Decisions are being made as more and more data are coming in. This explains why one medication was taken off the US market in October 2010 because of safety concerns. It should be wise to start these medications under a physician's supervision. Beware that some of the side effects may include changes in vision, dizziness, or drowsiness. Caution should be used if working with heavy machinery or driving, especially in the first few days due to the possible changes to vision and impairment of muscle movements.

Besides the short list of medications submitted here, there are instances in which the doctor may prescribe some other medications for the same purpose. This falls into the category of "off-label" use. This expression simply means that a physician can use a medication that is prescribed to treat a different condition—for example, a medication known to treat seizures may be used to address numbness and tingling in the legs and hands (neuropathy) of a patient. The doctor can also combine two medications for a diagnosis or use the prescribed medicine beyond the recommended time period. Dialogue and clear communication is always important in the doctor-patient relationship.

While addressing the issue of medication for weight loss, there is a list of over-the-counter medications as well as a few herb-based products that are offered as an alternative to FDA-approved medications. Their use is up to the patient. In most cases, there is no scientific evidence to support the claims made by homeopathic remedies. We must be aware that some of these products can be linked to serious medical conditions. One of the dilemmas of using these natural remedies is a lack of supporting scientific data and inability to know the proper dosage. At any rate, please use prudence and good judgment to stay healthy and fit.

## Vagus Nerve Blockage

Among those who are struggling with obesity, what happens to the people who have tried almost everything under the sun, short of surgery, with no satisfactory result? Indeed, after trying the diet and exercise approach with no proven sustained benefit, many venture into medications. But often, they have to stop because of different unacceptable side effects and regaining lost pounds. These people may contemplate bariatric surgery; however, they are not sure of the outcome and they fear the eventual complications. These people should take a look and be considered for Vagus nerve blockage (vBloc). This procedure is recommended for adults with a BMI between thirty-five and forty-five who have failed to show appreciable improvement under supervised qualified weight-management services. It is associated with other significant comorbidities, including hypertension and DM. The FDA approved the vBloc with the Maestro Rechargeable System (EnteroMedics, St Paul, MN) to treat obesity. The vBloc functions as a pacemaker-like device. Placed laparoscopically at the gastroesophageal junction, it sends intermittent electrical signals to the Vagus nerves. It does not change the gastrointestinal anatomy, yet it can produce a durable measurable result with a decreased risk of complications seen in bariatric surgery.[16]

---

16 Apovian C. M., S. N. Shah, B. M. Wolfe, et al., "Two-Year Outcomes of Vagal Nerve Blocking (vBloc) for the Treatment of Obesity in the ReCharge Trial." *Obes Surg.* Published online August 10, 2016. www.endocrineweb.com/professional/obesity/obese-patients-achieve-sustained-weight-loss-vagus-nerve-blockade.

## Surgery

You must have heard before that surgery to lose weight should be a last resort. We must admit there are instances when despite diet, physical activity, and medication, people may be advised or need to opt for surgery. Again, there are different strokes for different folks. The NIH recommends that surgery can be considered for a patient with morbid obesity whose BMI is above forty, or if the patient has serious medical issues with a BMI greater than thirty-five, if such an intervention would improve the patient's condition. The overall increase in obesity has also contributed to an increase in the number of people opting for surgery. It is reported that there is an average of more than two hundred thousand surgeries performed annually, costing more than $6 billion a year. Usually such a patient does not benefit from any other means of weight loss, and dieting alone has failed. The role of surgery is to physically intervene and limit the stomach space, thereby reducing the amount of food and calories taken in. Because surgery tends to bypass or reduce part of the small intestine, it also reduces the intake in calories and nutrients for the body.

Surgical interventions that are performed (gastric bypass, adjustable gastric banding, and vertical-sleeve gastrectomy) fall under the title of bariatric surgery. This is a serious intervention during which the size of the stomach is restricted and digestion goes much slower, or a part of the digestive system is removed or bypassed to reduce food absorption, thereby decreasing calorie absorption. The Lap-Band procedure, also called laparoscopic adjustable gastric banding, has become quite popular, as it is less invasive and reversible. It consists of surgically inserting a silicone/prosthetic adjustable band that constricts the stomach and makes the patient feel full much earlier than usual with less amount of food. Such a procedure can be adjusted based on needs and symptoms to meet the set goal. It usually consists of making a few tiny cuts around the stomach, then after distending the stomach with carbon dioxide, the surgical instruments are inserted through those tiny cuts; with the help of a camera, the surgeon performs the procedure laparoscopically while watching it on a video. He wraps a silicone band around the stomach and then seals it securely. The whole procedure is done within twenty to thirty minutes and costs an average of $22,000. Other common surgical procedures include the Roux-en-Y gastric bypass, in which the stomach is stapled with bowel rearrangement, and the sleeve gastrectomy, in which most of the stomach is removed and what is left is converted into a thin tube. With a smaller stomach, less food can be ingested. This approach is quite popular and provides appreciable weight reduction.

Surgical procedures entail having a permanent commitment to following a healthy lifestyle. Studies concur that such procedures do help people to lose weight and improve their overall medical conditions. The approach and the procedures keep evolving for better results. It is worth noting that surgical interventions as a means for weight loss are not benign. There are complications and secondary issues such as infections, leakage, bleeding, bowel blockages, blood clots, respiratory difficulties, and delayed healing process that can complicate the patient's condition during and after the procedures. This is not to be considered lightly. It requires a lifetime commitment to a modified diet with long-term implications. There are instances of blood clots in the lungs. The mortality risk one month after surgery is about two to five people among 1,000. Taken as a whole, the chance of dying can go as high as 2 percent, but this is improving with time. Patients may develop malabsorption and will need to be on lifelong supplementation. Before going forward with such an intervention, the patient usually needs medical, cardiology, and other specialists' clearance based on the patient's overall medical condition. Since more young people are considering surgical intervention, many questions and issues need to be addressed.[17] Many of the

17  Martin, Louis F., Obesity Surgery 1st Edition, McGraw-Hill, Medical Publishing Division.  https://asmbs.org/patients/bariatric-surgery-procedures. www.obesityaction.org.

long-term complications such as weight regain, strictures, hernias, ulcers, and nutrient deficiencies can be avoided if the patient adheres to the doctor's recommendations and close follow-up. The best surgical result occurs when it fits into a comprehensive, multidisciplinary approach that addresses the patient's lifestyle and commitment to behavioral changes.

Overall, when it comes to successfully managing overweight and obesity, the available tools include proper diet, supplements, regular exercise, behavioral modifications, drugs, and surgery. The approach is tailored to the individual's needs and condition.

# CHAPTER 13

## Facing the Challenge of the Weight-Loss Plateau

For one reason or another, you have decided to change or improve your diet and to be more consistent in your physical activity and your exercise schedule. As a result, you are very happy to notice that is it paying off. You are losing the extra weight. You are enjoying the number going down each time you step on the scale. So, you continue to eat right and exercise, and you feel great. This goes on for a few weeks. Then you notice that the scale stops budging. Things are not proceeding as expected. Although most of us expect it, somehow it still seems surprising that you have reached a point where you no longer lose any more pounds. Your weight loss has just suddenly stopped. This is what is called a weight-loss plateau.

Why did your success grind to a halt? There is a good reason for such a change. It is common to reach a point when the scale is not moving in the direction you want. As you lose weight, it becomes more difficult to lose more because our metabolisms slow down. Remember, our weights, the quality and quantity of foods, our levels of physical activity, and our BMIs all play a role in our metabolisms. When our weights go down, we lose some muscle mass (hence the need to exercise to maintain muscle mass), and our metabolisms slow down to adjust. Our bodies have been programmed to deal with "starvation" rather than excess, as previously mentioned. During the first weeks of our systematic healthy lifestyles, eating many fewer calories and burning more calories through exercise creates a deficit in energy to sustain the various functions of the body. The body goes to its bank of stored energy. This source of energy is called glycogen, and it is found in the liver and the muscles. As this type of carbohydrate (glycogen) is released to be spent and to compensate for the negative balance in energy, it is burned and water is released as well because glycogen is stored with water.

Initially, because your caloric intake decreases, the body must spend some of its glycogen storage to keep up with the new trend. There is a depletion of stored fat, and water is released. This results in an appreciable weight loss in the beginning. As a matter of principle, depending on body mass, our bodies consume at least two-thirds of the absorbed calories to keep all the necessary bodily functions going. Remember, we need a certain number of calories for breathing and keeping our hearts beating (BMR). As we exercise and keep down the number of calories consumed through our healthy diets by watching our portions and counting calories, our weights go down, our BMIs go down, and so do our BMRs. As our BMIs decrease, even if the percentage lost is the same, the number of calories burned is less in moving around at the same rate.

There is a constant dialogue between the brain and the body. Researchers, including some from Beth Israel Deaconess Medical Center, a teaching and research affiliate of Harvard Medical School, support the fact that the hypothalamus plays a key role in maintaining what is called the energy balance. Simply put, normally, based on genetics, the brain monitors changes in body weight and takes steps—among other things—on our satiety center to maintain equilibrium by increasing or decreasing our appetites. We also know now that the microbes in the gastrointestinal tract have an influence on obesity. These are influenced by the food we eat.

As the process of weight loss continues, signals are sent, and the body calls for adjustments to restore order.

This means the brain acts to restore the energy balance by secreting hormones. The body is adjusting and is consuming fewer calories. If we keep the trend of controlling calories through exercise and diet, our bodies reach a point at which it learns to use less calories (increased efficiency), leaving more extra calories to spare for the pending famine that it feels may be coming. This can result in feelings of hunger, which can be the body's attempt to counter weight loss by increasing intake. A glass of water helps!

## Eight Ways to Scale the Weight-Loss Plateau Barrier

First thing, do not be discouraged, and do not panic. Remember your initial goal and the reason you started such an endeavor. You may need to go back to the drawing board and see what needs adjustment. Simply put, you need to find ways to decrease your calorie intake further and burn more. Sometimes it may be necessary to stay at a certain weight for several weeks until the body's metabolism readjusts and does not think it is in starvation mode.

Here are a few steps to help you go beyond the stubborn wall hampering your progress:

1. Sometimes the initial calculation that leads us to the number of calories targeted to lose was

underestimated, or our way of counting our consumed calories is not adequate. For example, we count the cups and spoons of foods, but we may forget the so-called diet drink with its own number of calories or the salad dressing, the added condiments to our healthy plates, or the apparently innocent snacks we grab here and there. Everything must be accounted for. We need to remember that low fat does not mean zero calories. If you eat enough low-fat, low-calorie foods, they do add up.

2. Keep a careful record of everything that goes into your mouth, including gum, food and wine tasting, ice cream, sodas, butter, margarine, or even licking your child's lollipop.

3. Reassess how and what you eat at work, with friends, and in restaurants.

4. Revisit your diet and exercise plan. A little reshuffling and a tweak here and there may make a huge difference—for example, a different breakfast to begin the day, fewer sugary snacks, or a decrease in calories from carbohydrates and an increase in protein intake may have a significant influence. Also, make sure you are getting enough fiber and water. Increased fiber in the diet will increase satiety. The best sources are complex carbohydrates, fruits, and

vegetables. Eat more high-energy, low-calorie fruits and vegetables. Review the types and the schedule of physical activity and exercise you are getting.

5. Get a pedometer to keep track of your movement. It will make you more conscious of the need to move around indoors as well as outdoors. It will also boost your morale and encourage you when you see that you take thousands of steps each day.

6. You may decide to reduce your caloric intake further, increase your time spent in physical activity, and revisit all facets of your daily lifestyle. Remember, weight loss is depends on a combination of factors. Ultimately, you want to be healthy. Do not starve!

7. Review your overall environment and your daily routine. What has changed? What can be changed? How many hours are you sleeping? Are you more stressed than usual? Are you drinking enough water? What medications or supplements/natural products are you taking?

8. Revisit your initial weight-loss goal and compare it to where you are now. After losing ten, twenty, thirty, or forty pounds, do you want to continue to struggle to make it to your goal weight, or would it be healthier to maintain your current weight? Sometimes it is worth reassessing the situation

to see if your current weight is appropriate for your profile and personality. Depending on how heavy you were at the beginning, you may switch gears and work on a smooth transition to a new long-term lifestyle and to maintain what you have accomplished so far. Remember to revamp your eating habits and be self-conscious of the daily activities that will trigger some positive changes that are beneficial to your health. Because, after all, staying fit and healthy is a lifetime commitment. It is worth it if we want to have a healthy and enjoyable life.

# CHAPTER 14

## Keeping Obesity at Bay for Good

After a wake-up call about our weights, sometimes a recent medical diagnosis, we become more health conscious and take the necessary steps to have a healthier lifestyle. We are pleasantly surprised that it helps. Our clothes fit better, we have more energy, and we feel great. However, after moving the number down the scale, it would be a shame to add those pounds back on. Unfortunately, living long and staying healthy is a journey with twists and turns, but it must go on. We cannot afford to let down our guards and relinquish all our efforts in such an undertaking. As a matter of fact, we do not even want to think of the alternative. It is time to adopt a new mental and physical approach to stay the course of this lifestyle change.

Here are twelve steps to hold obesity at bay for good and maintain a healthy lifestyle:

## 1. Be fully committed and have a purpose in life.

All of us have heard this expression: "talk is cheap." This applies to health. We cannot stay healthy and fit by being passive and neglectful and continuing to ignore some basic rules of health. Actually, just by taking a few simple actions, we can appreciably improve our overall conditions.

When we have been diagnosed with a health condition, if we cannot change the condition, we still can have a positive influence on our overall quality of life. Like everything else in life, adopting a healthy lifestyle and getting rid of conditions such as overweight and obesity requires full commitment and perseverance. In fact, losing weight in a healthy manner can help with diabetes, cholesterol, heart disease, and blood pressure management. If there ever is a good addiction, staying fit and healthy should be it. However, being obsessed and excessive in anything becomes counterproductive. Seek ways to stay healthy: diet, exercise, stress and financial management, and even engaging in purposeful activities such as working or volunteering.

## 2. Develop healthy eating habits.

The USDA's "My Plate" provides a valuable model to help us keep a handle on our food intake. It is imperative to watch the quality and quantity of what we eat. Our calories should come from quality, low-fat, low-cholesterol foods such as a variety of fruits, vegetables, legumes, whole grains, vitamins, and minerals and limited sugars, salt, and fat.

Our snacks should be made up of fresh fruits, nuts, whole grains, and low-fat yogurt. We should eat an average of three regular meals daily. We should not skip meals. Because of mass foods production and all the processing steps that can strip foods of important nutrients, a multivitamin supplement may be needed, based on the diet and type of foods consumed. Caffeine and alcohol consumption should be limited. Smoking and doing drugs must be avoided at all costs. Stay away from crash fad diets because they do not help in the long run. They may cause more harm than good. Furthermore, dedicate time to plan and prepare your meals as well as your snacks. Keep away from unhealthy choices that may be tempting, especially when hungry or stressed out. It may be helpful to surround yourself with supportive people on a similar path to health.

## 3. Exercise regularly.

To stay healthy, diet and exercise go hand in hand. However, when mentioning exercise, some of us seem to be hesitant because of some physical ailments and logistical constraints. It is worth noting that being active is part of living. We may not be able to run marathons or engage in any professional sports. Nevertheless, it is paramount that we are engaged in some form of physical activity that may be just walking half an hour daily with our pedometers to keep track of movement and encourage us. We may even start one block at a time. We may also perform household chores that keep us physically active. Any physical activity is not only good for our bodies but also helps to keep a healthy brain.

## 4. Consult with your primary care doctor.

It is common sense for people to educate themselves, to work, to save and seek a decent, and secure life. Unfortunately, sometimes they work so hard they do not have time to take care of their bodies.   When it comes time to see a doctor, they tend to put it off until it is too late. This must not be so! To stay healthy, we must have a proactive approach. We need to focus on preventing disease and addressing any symptoms with our doctors immediately instead of waiting for issues to become urgent. To stay ahead of the game, we must have a physician with whom we keep a cordial relationship and one with whom we feel comfortable enough to discuss any medical concerns. A primary care doctor is not there to be seen only when we are sick. We should have regular, scheduled checkups and appropriate screenings based on our ages, our risk factors, and our overall medical conditions. If you are unhappy with one doctor, get another one. He or she should be competent, affable, and available.

## 5. Be cognizant about brain health.

Regardless of our chronological ages, all of us go through the aging process. We should not only be mindful about maintaining ourselves in excellent physical shape, but we must also be mindful that longevity is more enjoyable if we conserve our cognitive abilities. To stay fit, diet and exercise will help, but we must also engage in activities that stimulate our brains and keep us sharp. Reading, solving crossword or jigsaw puzzles, acquiring new knowledge and new skills, and pursuing difficult tasks and assignments will feed the brain and keep it healthy. Stimulate the brain through pleasant activities and relationships. Meditation, relaxation, and spirituality also help the mind and the body.

"The brain matters" is an integrative approach in which everything, every aspect of life, is taken into consideration to enable a person to conclude what is needed and to use his or her conviction to make the appropriate changes for the desired lifestyle with support and counseling. This is also viewed as "mind-body medicine".

## 6. Nurture your education.

Acquiring knowledge and wisdom must continue to be our top priority. We must continue to teach people how to eat right, what foods to choose, and how to cook healthy foods without violating their social and cultural values, or their "soul food." Therefore, all of us should focus on educating the population as to what will keep them healthy and giving them motivation to change their behaviors. People need to turn away from sodas and sugary drinks and develop a taste for clean and fresh water. The government should also take steps to preserve the potability of water.

## 7. Enjoy being and staying alive.

For many, this may sound like a given. Nevertheless, we may go through the motions of living without being fully involved in life. What does this mean? Life must go on with a sense of purpose for everyone. All of us have our place under the sun. Therefore, we must have plans and pursue them. We must also be equipped to face the challenges. The secret is in our overall attitudes about the difficulties we encounter throughout our existence. We need to master our emotions and not be mastered by our emotions, our moods. The proper attitude helps us to forgive and forget, to hold no grudges and not be vindictive. The right attitude helps us to manage stress appropriately, communicate efficiently, and navigate through life with no more than our proper share of trouble. Do not take everything seriously all the time. Engage in activities you can enjoy. Laughter is good medicine.

## 8. Be mindful of relationships.

We are not a bunch of isolated islands. We need to interact. To do so efficiently, we must respect certain rules and boundaries. We have our place among family members, friends, coworkers, and community members. Family and friends keep us connected and help us to stay involved and interested in what is going on around us. Researchers support the fact that balanced relationships are good for our well-being. We need to have fun, laugh, be sociable, enjoy vacation time, travel, walk, write, create art, and play music. It is good for our health.

## 9. Keep an eye on our financial conditions.

In movies, everyone is always spending money and getting the coolest new gadget. In reality, though, our personal financial conditions may not be as wonderful as the people on TV. This also plays an important part in our health status. Although money cannot buy life, it can affect the various treatments of our medical conditions. There is a correlation between our financial situations and our health conditions. Several studies support the fact that higher-income people generally enjoy a healthier and much longer life. We need to take steps as early as possible to develop a stable financial condition to meet our basic needs, live in better neighborhoods, and face unforeseen events. This may require financial expertise that we do not have. It is not a bad move to learn early and to consult financial experts to develop the proper portfolio for long-term financial stability. At any rate, the basic rule remains—not only to live within our means and avoid mortgaging our futures and the futures of the younger generation by accumulating debts, but also to manage to have a 10 to 20 percent savings from our revenues. We should also contribute to our communities and other worthy cause and help society. After all, no one lives only for himself. If these things were not done before, it is time to start now.

## 10. Watch the company we keep.
Some of the friends we have may make us worse off than declared enemies. We must not allow others to impose tasks on us. We may not be able to do anything about our families, but friends are freely chosen. We need to

surround ourselves with people who give us good advice, who can calm us down when we lose our tempers, who are brave enough to give us the right advice even though we may strongly object. We need to be with people who are pleasant and truthful, who have values and ethics, and who can distinguish right from wrong. This is not to say that we should avoid all burger eaters or carnivores. This is merely saying we should be aware of the company we keep and choose friends wisely. It will make a difference in our stress levels, our sleep health, and many other aspects of our lives, including our weights and our overall successes. Our friends and family have a large effect on our behaviors and what we eat. As the saying goes, "Tell me who your friends are, and I will tell you who you are."

## 11. Be mindful of social and physical environments.

To stay healthy, we must acknowledge the well-established correlation between health status and living condition. Our health can be adversely affected by substandard housing conditions with things such as pest infestation, lead paint, dust, mold, and indoor allergens. Certain cities are toxic with pollution and hazardous materials. People in certain communities may have less access to healthy foods or safe places for exercise, and there may be a lack of proper schools or employment opportunities or even libraries. These kinds of environments are not conducive to healthy, long, and prosperous lives. Therefore, There must be a conjugated effort from the state, the community, and the people in such conditions to take steps to improve the quality of their lives, through education, behavioral changes, "safety net" measures, etc, and above all an individual determination to improve one's condition as much as possible.

## 12. Be prepared for unforeseen events.

After doing everything that is within our power to remain healthy, there are things that are beyond our control. That should not throw us off. If we do not take a proactive approach, things may get worse. We can always find comfort in knowing that we did everything that was within our power. Life can present unexpected setbacks. We do not wish them upon ourselves, but we are to be mindful of their possibilities. This is why we need to cultivate healthy relationships with our family members, our friends, and our acquaintances so they can support us in our times of need, when those times do come.

## Beware of the Side Effects of a Healthy Diet

Our bodies are sensitive to change—the bad ones as well as the good ones. When we make the decision to change course and adopt healthy eating habits along with exercise, the results are always rewarding. Nevertheless, our bodies may need some time to adjust. With a new diet, a new menu, and a change in eating habits, be prepared to encounter some temporary inconveniences. These may include stomach cramping, increased hunger and cravings, as well as some changes in muscle mass and skin tone, generalized malaise and fatigue, irritability, constipation, and other symptoms. Again, the reason is simple—the body is trying to adjust to the changes that are occurring. The discomfort is not going to last for long. The intensity and the extent are different for everyone. To cope with these variations, drink a lot of water and keep healthy snacks nearby. Stick with your diet, watch the company you keep—especially at the beginning—and keep a positive attitude. It may be temporarily dark, but dawn is at hand. Stay the course. Experiences may vary, but at any rate, we must keep our eyes on the ultimate trophy.

In summary, after all is said and done, being overweight and obese is not insurmountable or even necessary. In fact, whether it is inherited or acquired, obesity can be prevented by the following:

1. Learning and finding ways to appreciate and encourage yourselves
2. Realizing you are wonderfully made ant not letting anyone or anything to convince you otherwise
3. Becoming aware of the predisposition for obesity early enough and acquiring adequate knowledge about it
4. Discovering weight gain early on and make changes immediately
5. Deciding to watch portion size
6. Eating regularly and not completely skipping breakfast
7. Preparing your own food when possible, including different meals and snacks
8. Dedicating at least half an hour daily for exercise
9. Having a friendly, positive attitude
10. Networking and communicating with others about successes, failures, and worries
11. Remembering you are humans and stop competing, or comparing yourselves with others.
12. Realizing that some issues and events are beyond your control, so you must live life fully on a daily basis and appreciate that there will be barriers to behavior change
13. Forgiving and holding no grudges

14. Reviewing sleep habits
15. Getting a handle on your stress level, not being a workaholic, and learning to relax and enjoy life
16. Being a decent, law-abiding citizen

# CHAPTER 15

## Food for Thought

### Personal Insights

Although obesity has recently become a worldwide concern, this issue has been tormenting us since the dawn of history. However, currently, it is easier to pass judgment than to effectively find a remedy. In fact, in harmony with the Epicurean philosophy—whether we admit it or not—all of us are seeking pleasure, satisfaction, and happiness as our ultimate goal. Eating does play a role in providing pleasure. Just think about your favorite dish or dessert, and your mouth is already watering. All of us love the aroma, the taste, and the ambiance of special, well-prepared, and well-seasoned foods. If you think about it, right now you can smell the spices in your favorite pasta dish or baked good. That is just human nature.

Therefore, it is not surprising that most of us forget the main role of food: to feed and to provide nutrients, fuel, and energy for our bodies to aid in staying active and performing various tasks. To make matters worse, for some people, food is cheaper than other recreation, and it is one of the major sources of pleasure that they can afford. They like the taglines in the advertisements to "have it your way" or "you deserve a break today." Often, the type of food we go after is saturated with fat, salt, sugar, and even chemicals. We are taking advantage of all the comforts that science and technology have provided us, such as trolleys, bikes, cars, tractors, televisions, phone apps, Internet, video games, as well as microwaves, diet pills, and elective surgery. However, the results of such a comfortable lifestyle may indeed make us physically ill.

We have reached a point in history when we have become prisoners of our appetites. Our desires seem to have smashed our willpower. Our lives revolve around appetizing food that is well seasoned with salt, butter, sugar, and spicy condiments. Our palates are flattered, and we become addicted to eating unhealthy foods. How many times do we eat just because the food is there and not because we are hungry?

## Managing the Pandemic of Obesity

To deal with the pandemic of obesity, we need to recognize that eating in itself is not evil. It is legitimate, and it is OK, but we must know what and how much to eat and drink and what to avoid. It needs to be done with moderation. We must learn to tame our appetites while becoming more physically active. A change of attitude is in order. It is human nature to be attracted to what is forbidden, hoping that we will not have to face the consequences. However, the consequences have already befallen all of us.

Going through a crash, restrictive diet for a few weeks or months will *not* do the trick. There must be a complete reeducation as to what and how much to eat and when to eat, while respecting the fact that people are different. What works for one person will not necessarily work for another one. Give yourself time and space. Be willing to adjust. Seek assistance, if necessary, and persevere.

Here is an example of a healthy diet that may help you get rid of those extra pounds and burn those nasty calories:

**Breakfast:** Make a smoothie by putting in a blender a couple of fruits, vanilla or peppermint extract, or other healthy ingredients. You may vary the fruits for different flavors daily—apples, carrots, beets...you get the idea! A bowl of oatmeal or whole-grain cereal or a can of low-salt tomato juice is also good. A high-protein breakfast is better for most people (an egg, cheese, or fish). The bottom line is that it needs to be healthy and not require too much time to prepare.

**Lunch:** A salad is always a nice touch at lunch. If you cannot stand uncooked veggies, perhaps add some steamed vegetables, quinoa (has more protein than most grains but is not a high-protein food), and a fruit. Try to get as much of your daily intake of fruits and veggies off your checklist because by the time you get home, you will be too tired to cut vegetables. (It also helps to prepare lunch the night before!)

**Dinner:** Find some fish you like and try to have it twice a week. Fish are filled with omega-3 and will aid you on this journey to health and even improve your mood. There are so many species of fish out there! Make sure to check the quality and quantity.

**Snacks**: Healthy snacks include one-quarter cup of nuts, two tablespoons of hummus, and a smidgen of crackers, fruits, and plain yogurt. These are things to look for before grabbing that box of cookies, candy, or a piece of cake. My daughter used the excuse "at least Oreos are vegan." Whether they are marked low fat, organic, or healthy, you might still want to be careful with fried foods or decadent sauces. Do go for steamed or baked foods (non-fried, greasy foods). Do read ingredients and nutrition labels; do not be fooled by front-of-the-package claims!

Note: look at the serving size on the label. The calorie number on the box may not be for the whole box! Moreover, remember that you do not need to clean your plate! Yes, I know it seems wasteful when parts of the world struggle with scarcity. However, it is better to learn what portion size you will eat than to stuff your face and gain weight.

Drink more water before and between but not during meals. Stay active and be positive.

Here are some typical activities that help burn calories: walking, dancing, jogging, swimming, stretching, cycling, hiking, climbing stairs, gardening, and even taking care of daily errands or chores. I must confess I hate doing housecleaning. Nevertheless, one day, a guest called about a quick visit. I was the only one at home, and I had to clean up my mess. In two hours, I swept, mopped, and cleaned the house. By the time I was done, my aches and pain meant nothing compared to the pleasant surprise I had—according to my pedometer, I had burned close to 1,500 calories. I am not saying it would happen all the time, but daily chores do help burn calories.

## Be Proactive

It is OK if you fail to stick with the diet all the time. If you wish to have two pieces of red velvet cake for Valentine's day or some ice cream cake on your birthday, do not be so hard on yourself. Do not feel guilty or so beat up that you want to give up completely. We all need to be able to treat ourselves every now and then. However, we can no longer make it a habit to eat carelessly on a daily basis. Once we see the light, we ought to walk in it.

Purge! Remove from your grocery list, from your refrigerator, your freezer, your kitchen, or even your dining room certain categories of foods; that way, you will not be tempted at home because bad foods are not around. If you are diabetic and told by your doctor to avoid eating mangoes or candies—do not horde mangoes or candies. Simply do not buy them to give to the neighbor's kids! No excuses, please!

Go ahead! Get rid of those drinks, those cookies, those cakes, and that whole family of unhealthy foods and snacks. Pause right now, if you can, and start the purge. Replace them with apples, carrots, beets, watercress, spinach, broccoli, lettuce, strawberries, blueberries, and water. Before going to the grocery store, have your shopping list. Another good idea is not to go when you are hungry if you wish to avoid impulse buying. Identify some healthy ways to celebrate any upcoming special occasions without indulging in a giant Dairy Queen Blizzard every single holiday. Remember, if you plan your meals, you are much more likely to make healthy choices.

Lead by example. Badgering people is not your job. Because you are getting healthier does not mean you need to strong-arm others into joining you. Learn to say no without being cocky or self-righteous. If you are invited to a party, remember where you are going. Eat with moderation and choose what you put on your plate (quality and quantity). Do not go there with your little brown bag and tell everyone with a long face, "I can't eat this or that; I am on a diet." If you want to completely avoid a dish, just say that you are not hungry or you do not like it. Be natural and pleasant. If what is available is not against your religious beliefs or values, then take some with moderation. Remember to be sociable. A real diet should make you seem livelier with a healthy glow, not surly and judgmental. You want people to ask you how you manage to look so good Being healthy does not necessarily mean being skinny.

Physical appearance alone does not necessarily reflect health. Looking slim and sexy is not a medal signifying excellent health. The real reason behind avoiding obesity is avoiding the eventual diseases and complications that arise from it.

Suffice it to say that while we are taking care of the insides, our appearance should also be well cared for with proper hygiene and attire. This should be taken into consideration to present a general positive view of ourselves.

Not all obese people have medical ailments, but the risk is higher for obese people than for the general population. Throughout history, there have been instances in which obesity was favored. There are still some regions in the world, even some parts of the most modern countries, where being plump is an asset, a sign of prosperity, happiness, good health, and even fertility for women. But research and scientific data prove it is not conducive to health and longevity. In fact, studies have shown that calorie restriction may be associated with longevity.

Diet is not the scapegoat for obesity. It is not the sole cause! Weight does not depend exclusively on your diet. An anthropological approach is needed, meaning taking into consideration all the aspects of human life, including genetic, physical, anatomical, epidemiological, economical, biological, physiological, behavioral, environmental, political, individual, familial, educational, social, and cultural aspects of life. It requires an interdisciplinary approach.

If obesity persists with genetic adjustment and human transformation, is it possible that most of the world's population will become obese? If so, will that become the norm? Will we be forced to realign our values and change the BMIs? Must we leave everything at the mercy of Mother Nature to put everything back in order? Will we give rise to another definition of the phrase "survival of the fittest"?

Here is another approach to win the war against obesity:

1. Be aware of the urgency of this condition and its effects. View it as a serious issue that needs to be

tackled immediately. Do not say, "I will wait 'til I'm thirty or forty-five to deal with this." Start early. Start today!

2.  Realize that everyone is different and unique. It is not a competition. Friends and family members may find that they do compete a little with each other in certain areas of their lives. However, when it comes to weight management, do not quit just because you are not losing as much weight as quickly as others. Everyone is different. As human beings, we need to realize there will be setbacks, but no matter what, we can never give up.

3.  Take charge by determining how much you need to lose based on age, gender, height, and body structure.

4.  Adopt a healthy, balanced diet, aiming to eliminate unhealthy foods and unhealthy habits. This means eating a diet high in fruits, legumes, vegetables, whole grains, and nuts and eliminating highly sweetened, empty-calorie drinks and replacing them with water, consuming an average of two to three liters of water daily.

5.  Accept behavioral modifications and acquire the proper knowledge to act constructively. If your partner raises his or her eyebrow when you reach

for Haagen-Dazs, note that he or she is merely trying to help you, not antagonize you.

6. Have a network of support. When disasters happen in your life and you want to sit and eat a whole tub of cookies and ice cream, that is the time to tap into your support network.

7. Remember that weight management is a long-term commitment that requires daily actions.

After all is said and done, recent data provide encouraging news. The ascending curve of obesity seems to have reached its peak among certain sectors of the population. Advances in research about how to find the most effective strategies to successfully manage obesity continue. With the commitment of the research, development, and scientific sectors, along with education and cooperation between private and public sectors, I am confident that we will definitely be able to handle obesity.

# CHAPTER 16

## Children and Obesity

Welcoming children into this world is one of the most rewarding experiences in life. It gives us satisfaction and pride as well as a heavy responsibility to shoulder. A newborn is going to live in this world and face countless numbers of challenges. Generally, parents want to shield the baby from many inconveniences or threats to his or her life. He or she is constantly showered with love and coddling. Instinctively, we want our babies to grow and be healthy. People tend to congratulate a mother with a chubby, adorable baby. There seems to be a general belief that a child should eat everything on the plate and consume as much fat as possible to grow big and strong; then as an adult, he or she can be concerned about diet.

In addition, the culture encourages adolescents to gain weight, especially if they want to participate in sports.

They feel pressure to eat more and to gain as much weight as possible. Then, when they reach their thirties, forties, or more, the person has to pay attention to weight and face the consequences. Although this has been a long trend, things have changed significantly.

The adorable, chubby baby today may become the obese adolescent with type 2 diabetes and many other complications tomorrow. Why? After becoming obese so early in life, many continue this trend later and often until the end of life.

Obesity is more difficult to manage in an adult who was obese as a child. US statistical data show nearly one in five school-aged children ages six to nineteen is obese; from ages two to nineteen, the percentage goes much higher at one in three. Moreover, the number of obese children continues to climb, especially among American Indians, non-Hispanic blacks, and Mexican Americans. In the past three decades, the percentage of obese children and adolescents tripled! The current numbers suggest that almost one-third of our children already fall into the obese category. Some even predict that 50 percent of the population will be overweight or obese by fifteen to twenty years from now. For some reason, there is a trend to overeat. It has become even more alarming when it concerns our precious children. This data is given not to be a prophecy but to urge people to take steps to avoid reaching numbers that are even more grotesque.

According to the WHO, "Childhood obesity is one of the most serious public health challenges of the twenty-first century. The problem is global and is steadily affecting many low- and middle-income countries, particularly in urban settings. The prevalence has increased at an alarming rate. Globally, in 2015 the number of overweight children under the age of five is estimated to be over forty-two million. Almost half of all overweight children under five lived in Asia and one-quarter lived in Africa."[18]

In 2011, more than forty million children under the age of five were overweight. Consider a classroom of twelve children; two of them would be obese. In terms of statistical data, one out of every six children gathered would be obese. Childhood obesity also has a major effect on health. It increases the child's risk of becoming sick or being unable to fight infection. It is especially difficult to combat when we add the environmental and psychosocial factors such as a sedentary lifestyle of playing video games and the easy access to chips and unhealthy snacks, as well as the

18 WHO, "Childhood overweight and obesity," Global Strategy on Diet, Physical Activity, and Health.
Ogden CL, Carroll MD, Lawman HG, et al. Trends in Obesity Prevalence Among Children and Adolescents in the United States, 1988-1994 Through 2013-2014. JAMA 2016; 315:2292.
Gulati AK, Kaplan DW, Daniels SR. Clinical tracking of severely obese children: a new growth chart. Pediatrics 2012; 130:1136.

lack of safety and stability of a community. Before long, we wind up with children who have diseases that used to manifest only among the adult population, including type 2 diabetes, high blood pressure, heart conditions, asthma, sleep apnea, cancer, and even stroke. These chronic diseases bring along a lifetime filled with all kinds of problems and even disabilities, and premature death.

## What Causes Childhood Obesity?

Childhood obesity worldwide has reached an alarming proportion. One reason is the early exposure to high-fat, high-calorie foods and sugar-sweetened beverages. The child starts very early consuming more calories than are spent. The accumulated balance has to be stored and ultimately makes the child fat. These children grow up with well-developed and expanded fat cells, along with a lack of the necessary micronutrients. As they get bigger, they consume only what is given to them, what they are exposed to, which is usually micronutrient-deficient, fatty, processed foods that are also consumed by their parents. Parents are oftentimes a child's earliest and only example to follow. In addition, in many communities where child obesity is very high, there is very limited opportunity for exercise due to a lack of safe play areas, lack of parental time, and prevalence of devices as distractors.

When the children go to school, they are likely to be exposed to the same types of foods low in unrefined plant ingredients. These foods supply a lot of calories, salt, and sugar, while the antioxidants, phytochemicals, and necessary vitamins and minerals are nowhere to be found. This triggers a weak immune system because of early deficiencies in important micronutrients. This can cause all types of diseases including neurological ones and affect the child's learning ability. Beside eating habits, other factors in childhood obesity include genetic predispositions, metabolic programming, endocrine disorders, social and individual factors, level of physical activities, sedentary lifestyle, and lack of sleep.

We should also mention that some medical conditions require the use of certain drugs that cause weight gain and obesity.[19] In general, there are certain medical reasons that can be associated with weight gain. They include, hypothyroidism ( underactive thyroid), Cushing's syndrome ( caused by high levels of the hormone cortisol, or use of steroid for long time, or tumor), menopause, the ageing process with loss of muscle and slowing of metabolism (taking longer to burn calories), Polycystic ovary syndrome (PCOS) (affecting ovarian functions), reten-

19  Johnson, Jeffrey, Lyle Booman, Journal of Managed Care & Specialty Pharmacy: Volume 2 Issue (1) 1996 Jan;2(1):39-47., https://doi.org/10.18553/jmcp.1996.2.1.39
https://www.cdc.gov/healthyyouth/obesity/facts.htm.

tion of fluid, causing edema, excessive amount of stress, depression (Dysthymia), ovarian or pituitary tumor, etc. Among the medications that can contribute to putting on weight, we can mention some antidepressants, antipsychotics medications, the diabetes medication, steroid treatment. antipsychotic drugs, also medications used hypertension, epilepsy, migraines, etc.[20]

If a child received inadequate prenatal care, this is an added assault against his or her overall well-being. If a child grows up in an environment where he or she will be less active and might be exposed to factors, products, and experiences that are not ideal for harmonious development, this also can be reflected by weight gain. This is why childhood obesity and overweight is of great concern.

In short, childhood obesity affects a person sooner or later and deeply influences the quality and the quantity of one's life.

## Advice to Parents

Babies are obviously unable to make proper food choices. It is paramount that parents show them the way. That consists of starting early in training the child to eat

---

20 www.nhs.uk/Livewell/loseweight/Pages/medical-reasons-for-putting-on-weight.aspx
www.healthline.com/symptom/unintentional-weight-gain
www.webmd.com › Diet & Weight Management ›

healthy by showing through word and deed how to adopt and maintain a healthy, balanced diet. In so doing, when the children grow up, they will have a pathway to follow. If they see that all the meals are bought from a fast-food restaurant, as adults, this pattern will continue.

The childhood obesity epidemic is a fight that requires the involvement and commitment of the private sector as well as public institutions. It is a national security priority because our nation needs healthy young men and women to defend and maintain our right to choose freely, to prosper, and to assure continuity in the pursuit of a great life, liberty, and happiness. To meet such a challenge, all our resources must be pulled together. This includes all the factors: politics, economics, sociocultural values, and education.

Families need to provide the proper milieu that encourages a healthy and balanced lifestyle. Daily servings of fruits and vegetables should be the norm. The adults must lead by example in adopting the proper eating habits that include homemade meals, fruits, vegetables, legumes, and quality beverages. Instead of rushing to a fast-food place to get junk food and a sugary drink, we need to find a healthy restaurant, preferably with a family-friendly setting. Furthermore, well-known fast-food restaurant should make an effort to provide and promote healthy choices at competitive prices.

Physical activity needs to be emphasized early both at home and in school. It should be part of a regular daily schedule at home and in school. This early training not only sets a trend for a different lifestyle, but it helps in shaping the endurance of the child's muscles. It makes the child feel good and energetic. The child may even want to pursue professional sports in the future. It sets habits that the child is likely to follow for the rest of his or her life. Children should be encouraged to walk, run, bike, swim, and play sports based on their physical and mental fitness while observing proper guidelines for safety. Physical activities provide a platform to interact with others, to broaden sociocultural horizons, and to become balanced and sociable.

In addition, wealth is not distributed evenly, and some of us are more fortunate than others. [21]However, healthy choices must be easily available in all communities and at a price that is affordable to all parents. Why should a school meal be unhealthy? Why should some fruits be hard to find and costlier than some junk foods found on every corner in certain neighborhoods? Everyone should have a right to healthy food. All of us need to band together to facilitate healthy habits that consist of nutritious meals

---

21  Centers for Disease Control and Prevention (CDC). Obesity prevalence among low-income, preschool-aged children--New York City and Los Angeles County, 2003-2011. MMWR Morb Mortal Wkly Rep 2013; 62:17.

and healthy beverages along with available gyms for all. The government should not dictate to people what and how much to buy, eat, or drink, but it can surely educate and provide some incentive and a safety net so that everyone can have access to the resources, and environments, and foods that lead to a healthy and sustainable life.

The proper diet requires the availability and the consumption of vegetables, fruits, legumes, and whole grains, as well as an increase in appropriate physical activities. Parents must remember the best way to teach and lead is by example. Overall, prevention is the best medicine. Investing in our children, the younger generation, is a sure way to make our country great.

# Epilogue

Congratulations! Together we have gone through the journey in saying good-bye to obesity. The most important part consists of reviewing and implementing what you have learned or reviewed. We also need to remember that knowledge in this domain continues to evolve; we must remain open minded and willing to learn and improve our health continuously. The key is to take it one step at a time, stay the course, and be prepared to get up if we ever fall. Let us not compete with ourselves or anyone else. Let us remember that any change toward a healthier diet and becoming more physically active will have a positive effect in both quantity and quality in our lives. In a time of stress, uncertainty, and economic restraints, a healthier population will also contribute to a stronger and more prosperous America.

Let us do it together. A slimmer and healthier America is a national security issue. A healthier world makes it safer and more enjoyable for all the inhabitants of this planet.

# About the Author

After having brilliantly completed the cycles of primary and secondary education, Jean Daniel François received formal education and graduated with degrees in administration, economics, finance, and theology. He holds a bachelor of science, a bachelor of theology, a master in pastoral studies, and a master in economics. He also studied medicine at New York Medical College in Valhalla, New York, where he received his doctor of medicine. He is pursuing his career as a neurologist in New York, where he resides with his wife, Jocelyne, and their two grown children, Jean Daniel and Sarah. He is known as a lecturer, a radio speaker, and a man of science as well as faith. Dr. François wrote this book about getting overweight and obesity under control because he wants to share his beliefs with his readers that he has gleaned from his personal experience, his observations, his multiple instances of research, and his relationships with his patients and from reading several books and articles on obesity. He has written several books to help people engage in a new course for a healthy and enjoyable life by making choices based on appropriate acquired knowledge. For further details, please visit www.prescriptionforasuccessfullife.com.

## SELECTED BIBLIOGRAPHY

Obviously, it is very difficult to remember or take into account all the books read, the documents consulted, and the advice received in writing any book, let alone a book on obesity. I am indebted to a long list of experts in this field. Unfortunately, I am not able to list and credit everyone who has been a significant source in helping me to write this book. Suffice it to say, I am grateful to all of them—those I remember as well as those whom I may omit. I am confident that in their generous hearts they will find room to grant me forgiveness. My sources include the following:

Breuss, Michael, and Debra Fulghum, *The Sleep Doctor's Diet Plan*.

Bay, G. A. "Medical Consequences of Obesity." *J Clin Endocrinol Metab*. 2004; 89: 2583–2589.

Cordain, Loren, *The Paleo Diet*.

Diehl, Hans, and Aileen Ludington. *Dynamic Living: How to Take Charge of Your Health*. Review & Herald Publishing Association. 2005.

Fuhrman, Joel. *3 Steps to Incredible Health!* Gift of Health Press. Flemington, New Jersey. 2011.

Granberg, Ellen. Various books, articles, and interviews regarding the issues of obesity and how to keep the weight off.

Levetin, Estelle and Karen McMahon, *Plants and Society.* Third edition. 2003.

Lieberman, Shari. *Glycemic Index Food Guide.* Square One Publishers. Garden City Park, NY 11040.

Pamplona-Roger, George D. *Foods that Heal.* Review & Herald Publishing Association. 2004.

Sardi, Bill. *The New Truth About Vitamins & Minerals.* Here & Now Books. San Dimas, CA 91773.

Yeager, Selene, and the editors of *Prevention Health Books.* Rodale Press, Inc. Emmaus, PA.

## OTHER USEFUL SOURCES

American Heart Association.

American Journal of Clinical Nutrition.

American Medical News.

American Obesity Association.

American Society for Bariatric Surgery.

Association for Coordination and Research in Obesity and Nutrition. This European group provides information on obesity research in Europe.

Association for Morbid Obesity Support.

Cancer Project, The. 5100 Wisconsin Ave., NW, Suite 400, Washington, DC 20016. 202-244-5038. www.CancerProject.org.

Centers for Disease Control and Prevention, National Center for Chronic Disease Prevention and Health Promotion, Nutrition and Physical Activity, Overweight and Obesity

Ebbeling, Cara B., Janis F. Swain, Henry A. Feldman, William W. Wong, David L. Hachey, Erica Garcia-Lago, and David S. Ludwig. "Effects of Dietary Composition on Energy Expenditure During Weight-Loss Maintenance." *JAMA*. 2012; 307(24):2627-2634. doi:10.1001/jama.2012.6607

Health Worldnet.

Huffington Post, The. Healthy Living.

Jensen M. D., D. H. Ryan, C. M. Apovian, et al. "2013 AHA/ACC/TOS Guidelines for the Management of Overweight and Obesity in Adults: A Report of the American College of Cardiology/American Heart Association Task Force on Practice Guidelines and the Obesity Society." *J Am Coll Cardiol* 2014; 63:2985.

Mayo Clinic. Health Information.

National Center for Research Resources.

National Institute of Diabetes and Digestive and Kidney Diseases.

National Center for Health Statistics. Health, United States, 2011: With Special Features on Socioeconomic

Status and Health. Hyattsville, MD. US Department of Health and Human Services. 2012.

National Institute of Diabetes and Digestive and Kidney Diseases, Health Information.

National Institutes of Health. "Classification of Overweight and Obesity by BMI, Waist Circumference, and Associated Disease Risks." Body Mass Index Table.

National Institutes of Health. Health Information: Weight Loss and Control.

National Institutes of Health, National Heart, Lung, and Blood Institute. "Disease and Conditions Index: What Are Overweight and Obesity?" Bethesda, MD. National Institutes of Health. 2010.

National Obesity Education Initiative, Aim for a Healthy Weight, Information for Patients and the Public.

*Obesity* journal.

Obesity Law and Advocacy Center. This is a law firm in San Diego, California, that specializes in legal issues in obesity.

Olshansky S. J., D. J. Passaro, R. C. Hershow, et al. "A potential decline in life expectancy in the United States in the 21st century." *N Engl J Med*. 2005; 352:1138.

Pool, R. *Fighting the Obesity Epidemic*. Oxford University Press. New York, NY. 2001.

Skinner A. C., and J. A. Skelton. "Prevalence and trends in obesity and severe obesity among children in the United States." 1999–2012. *JAMA Pediatr*. 2014; 168:561.

Support Groups and Counseling.

US Centers for Disease Control and Prevention.

US Department of Agriculture. Dietary Guidelines for Americans.

US Department of Health and Human Services, US Department of Agriculture. "Dietary Guidelines for Americans."

US Food and Drug Administration. FDA Consumer. A Consumer's Guide to Fats.

WebMD.

http://www.medicinenet.com/obesity.

www.nutritionandhealthconference.org.

Medweightlossclinics.com.

www.medicalnewstoday.com

www.cdc.gov/obesity/childhood/basics.html

www.health.gov/dietaryguidelines/2010.asp

www.cdc.gov/physicalactivity

http://www.news-medical.net/life-sciences